MAKEUP
BY LIZ
KELSH

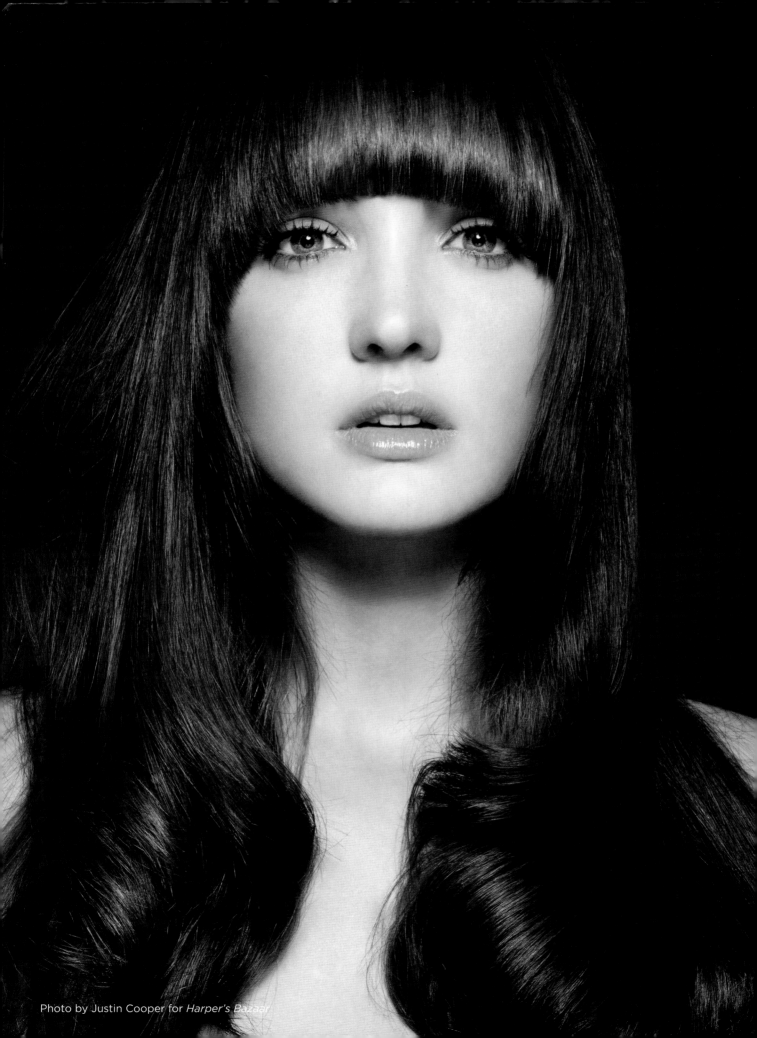

Photo by Justin Cooper for *Harper's Bazaar*

MAKEUP

BY LIZ KELSH

HarperCollins*Publishers*

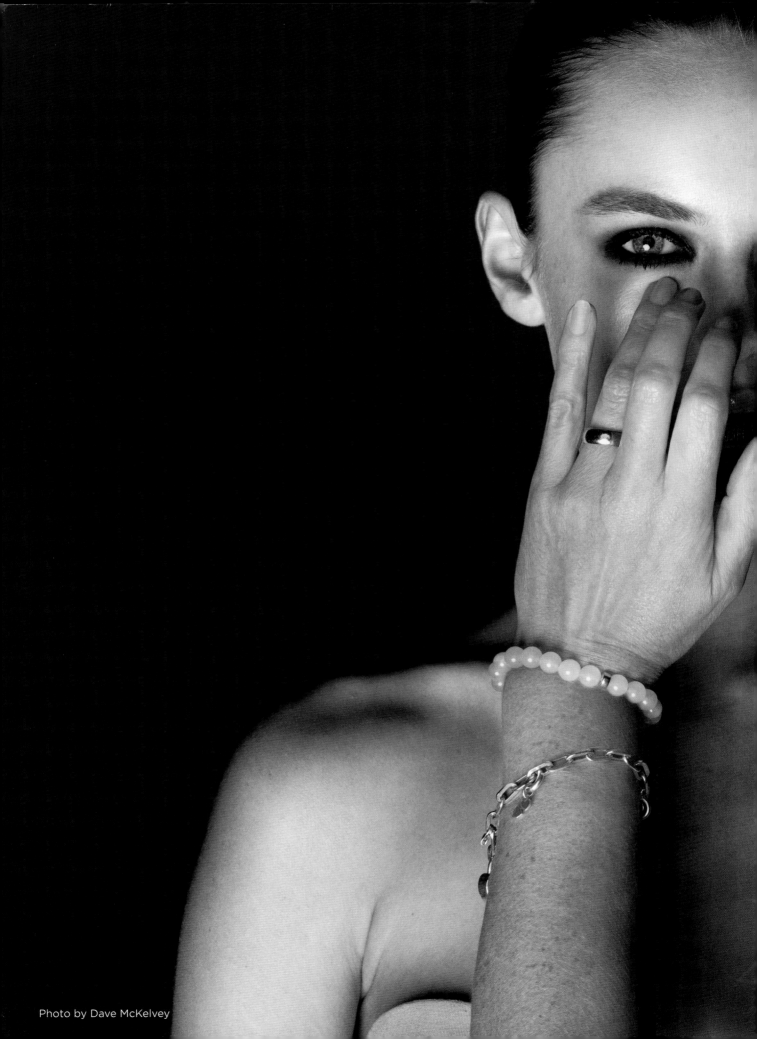

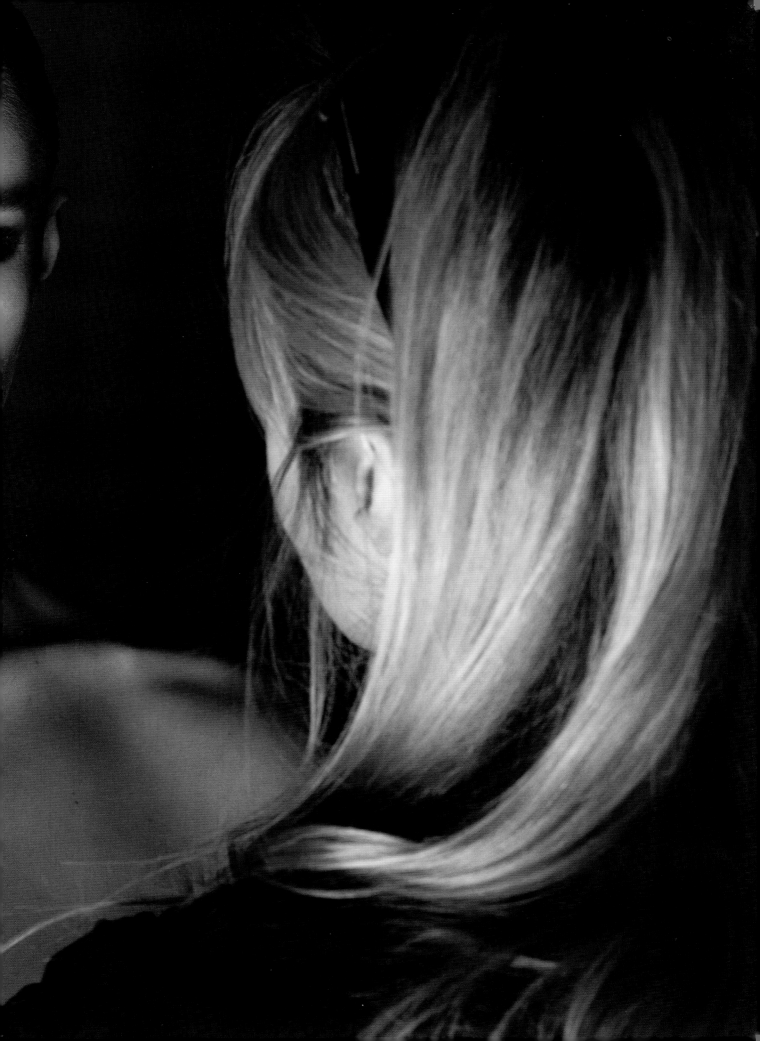

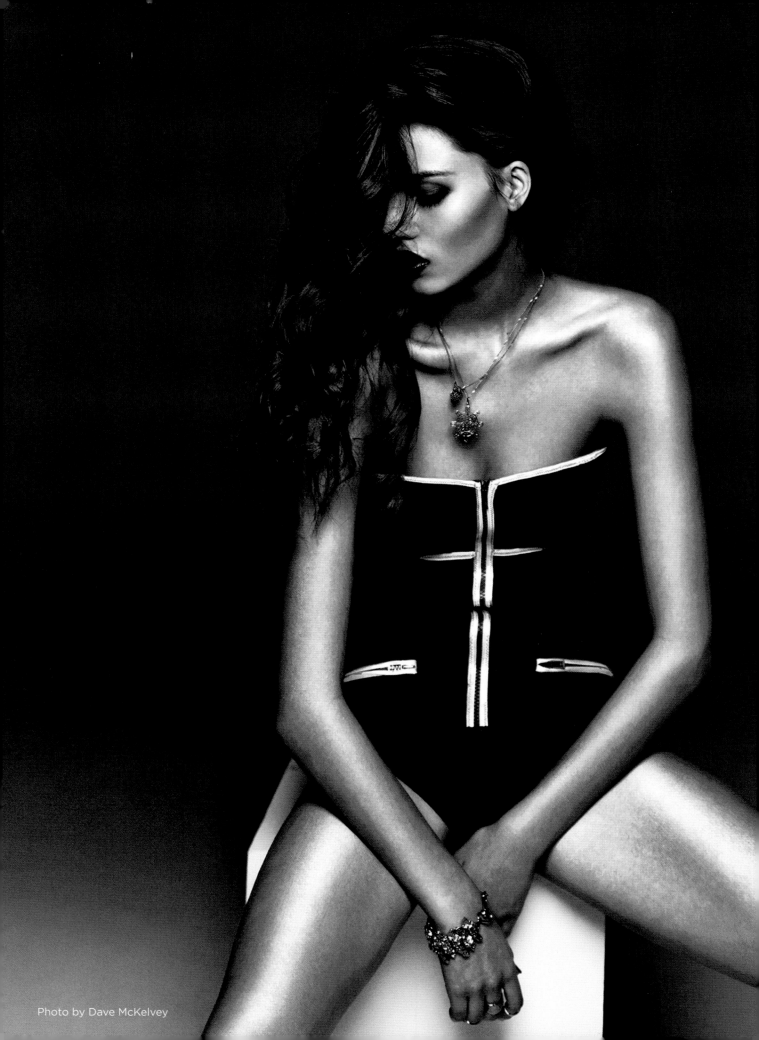

To all the beautiful women I've worked with and who have inspired me, especially my mum, my sister and, most of all, my gorgeous daughter, Ava.

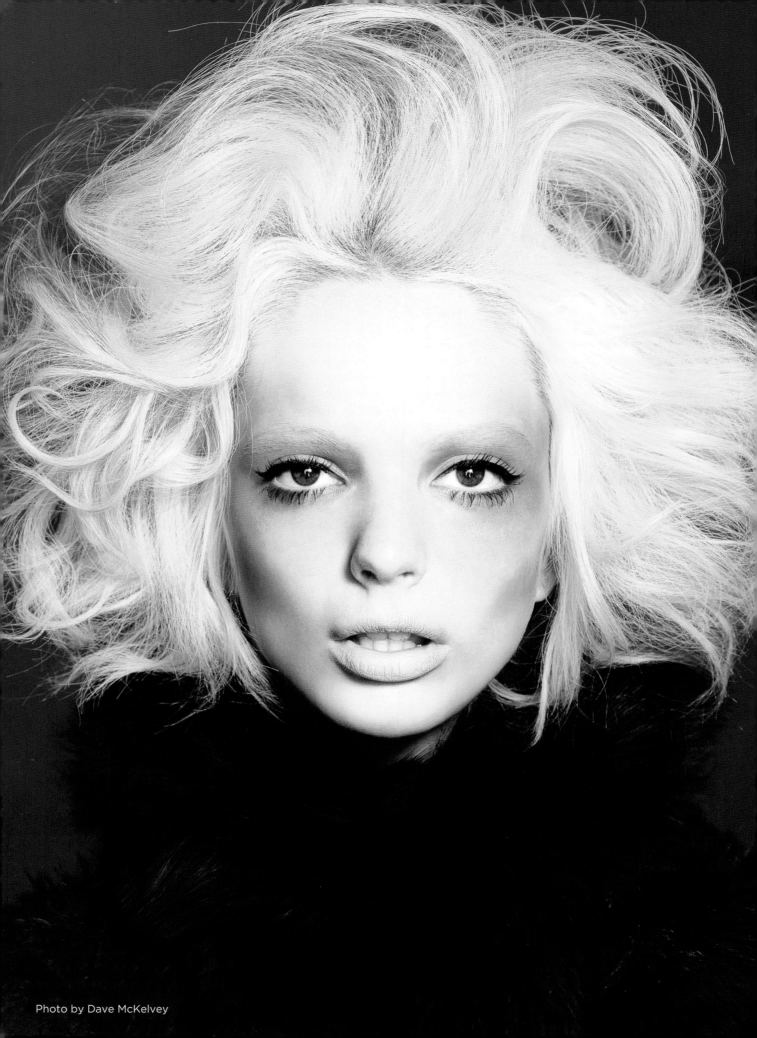

Photo by Dave McKelvey

Contents

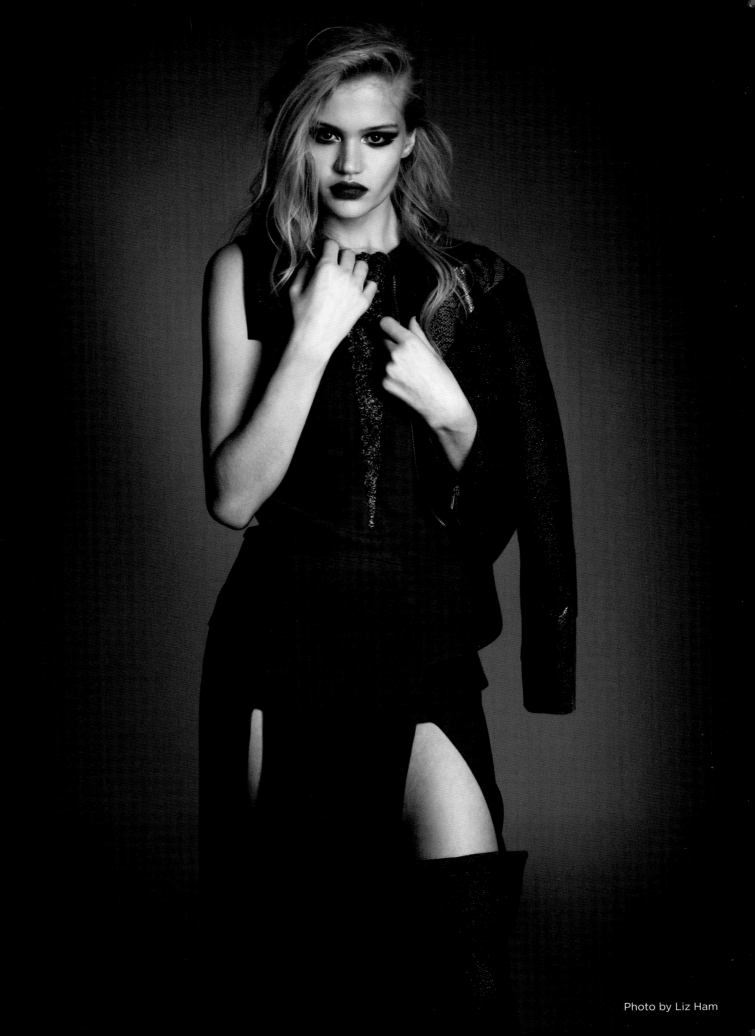

Photo by Liz Ham

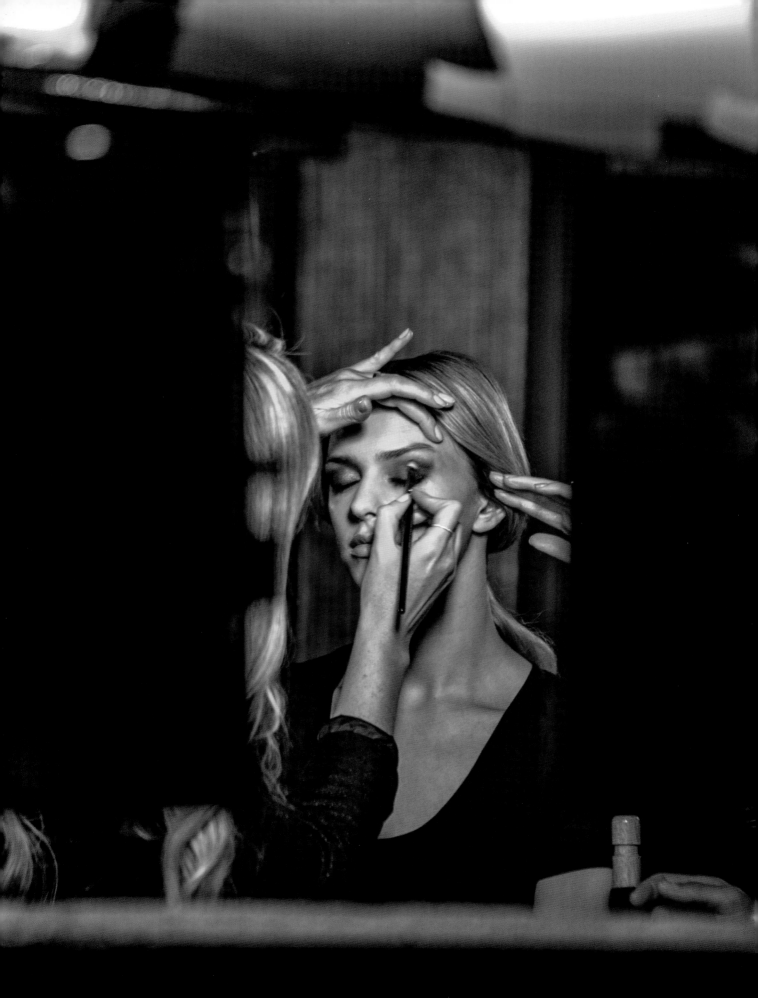
Photo by Liz Kelsh

Introduction

*Everything has its beauty
but not everyone sees it*

— CONFUCIUS (C. 551 – C. 479 BCE)

*The magic of makeup is that it makes
your beauty visible to everyone*

— LIZ KELSH 2014

I've been a makeup artist for a long time, and my mantra has always been that everyone is beautiful, but makeup makes them even more so. I see beauty in every face and love the power that makeup has to polish that beauty to the max and allow it to shine through. Light and colour can transform a face and I've always approached my art from this powerful perspective. Before starting a job, I observe the face, noting where the light reflects and the shadows fall, as well as the relationship between the features — do the brows need more definition? Is the jawline too soft? It is all about balancing the face.

I am a graduate of the school of trial and error. I experimented on anyone and everyone who would sit still long enough to have false lashes applied. I've been obsessed with makeup my entire life and feel fortunate to have made it my career. I've worked with some of the world's most beautiful women, including Nicole Kidman, Cate Blanchett, Naomi Watts, Miranda Otto, Jennifer Hawkins, Rihanna, Jennifer Aniston, Salma Hayek and Rose Byrne. I often get asked on photo shoots, 'what's the trick to this?', or 'how do you apply that?' or 'where are the apples of the cheeks?' and I get great pleasure from passing on my makeup know-how.

Almost every woman wears makeup but not many have been shown how to use it correctly. I love the *ahhhh* moment, when I show someone how to apply mascara correctly and how much more impact it has, or the confidence a groomed brow can bring, and that's what inspired me to write this book. I want this book to be all about you. I want to give you the tools, knowledge and confidence to be your own makeup artist.

The

Essentials

Skincare

The skin is the body's largest organ. It's the first to show the signs of sickness or poor diet, and it's also the first to show the signs of ageing. In this chapter I'd like to make sure your skincare routine is age-appropriate.

Tip

Drink plenty of water daily. Your skin will thank you for it.

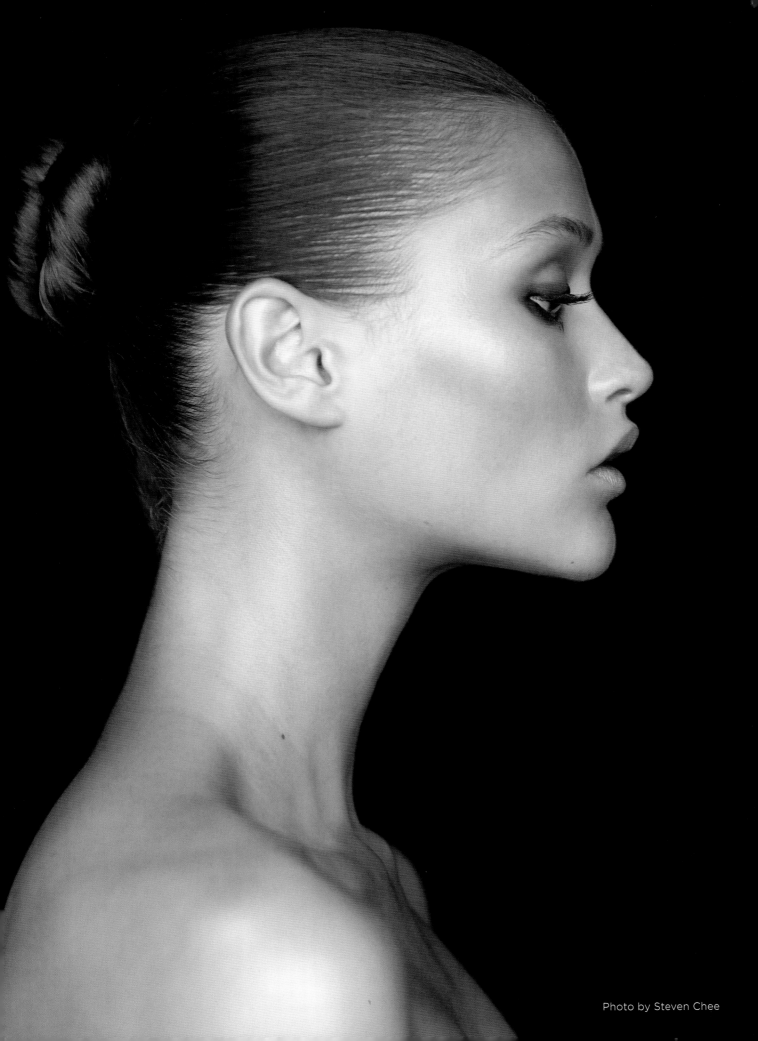

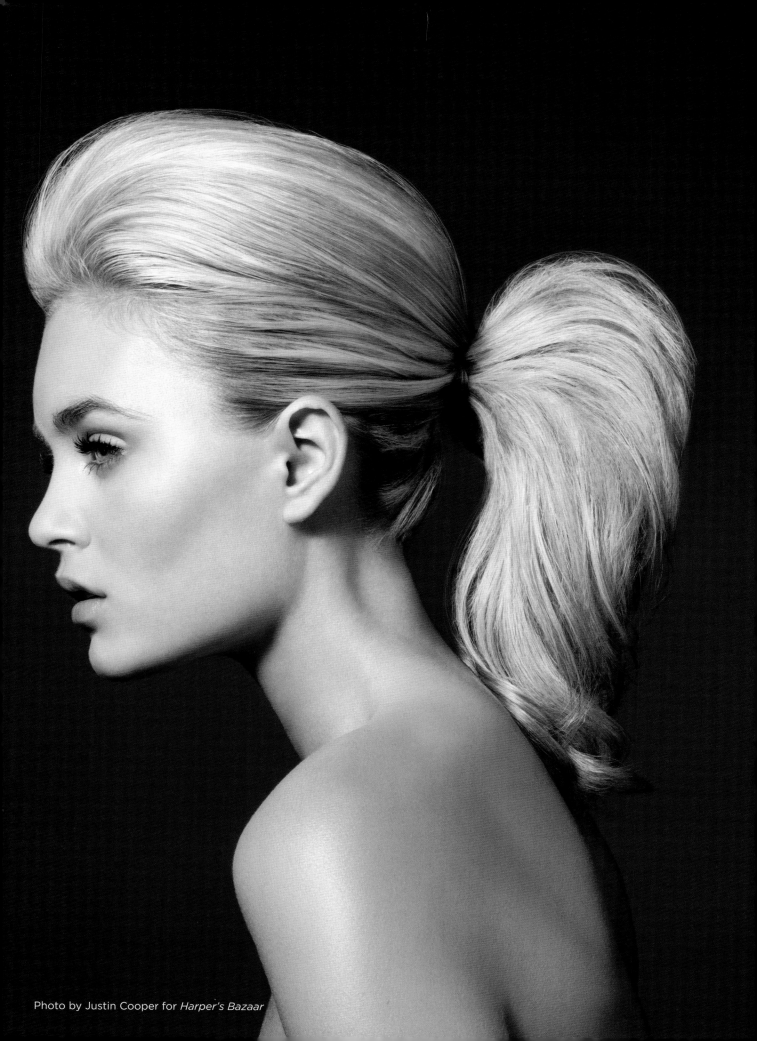

Photo by Justin Cooper for *Harper's Bazaar*

20s skin

I often find girls in their 20s either want to do too much or not enough when it comes to their skincare regime. In your 20s, it's all about KIS — Keeping It Simple. Try using a foaming cleanser in the morning and remember to double cleanse at night because this helps keep breakouts at bay. If you do suffer breakouts, add a treatment cream containing salicylic acid to your routine. Also, apply a combined SPF50 sunscreen and moisturiser daily — come rain, hail or shine — to slow down the effects of ageing. And if you are not already doing so, now is the time to start lifelong good habits: eating a balanced diet and undertaking regular exercise.

30s skin

Now is the time to up the ante with gentle exfoliation once or twice a week. Your skin's natural exfoliation cycle is half as efficient as it was in your 20s. Also, switch to a cream cleanser — it's less drying than a foaming one. Again, apply a combined sunscreen and moisturiser daily. A night cream containing retinol will help improve the tone and texture of your skin.

Tip

Wear a hat to the beach — it's the best anti-ageing tool available.

40s skin

The exfoliation process slows even more in your 40s, with sluggish dead cells sapping your skin of its natural glow. Exfoliation needs an extra boost, so switch to a chemical exfoliant to help break down the glue that holds onto the dead skin cells. Skin dehydration is also a concern at this age, so try a hyaluronic acid serum — it will do wonders. And remember the essential combined SPF50 sunscreen and moisturiser daily.

50s skin

The 50s approach is pretty much a continuation of the 40s. A good diet and regular exercise are great for skin of all ages — keep them going! And it goes without saying that you should drink plenty of water.

Tip

Exfoliate regularly. Your skin will look more luminous, foundation will last longer and skincare creams will be more effective.

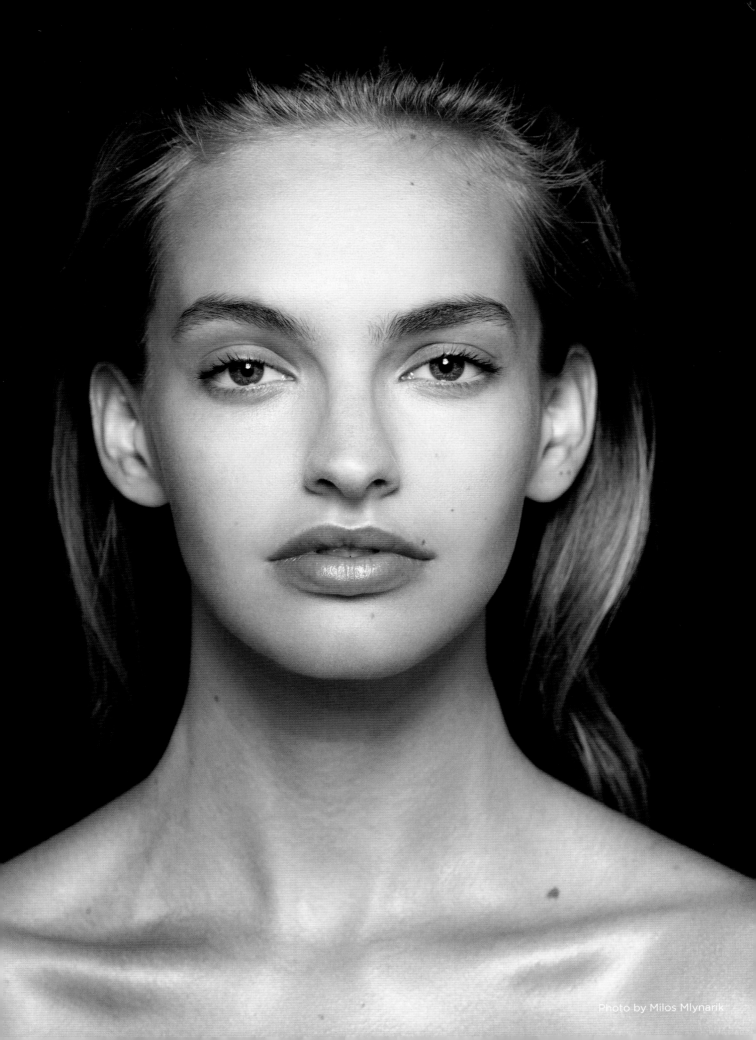

Photo by Milos Mlynarik

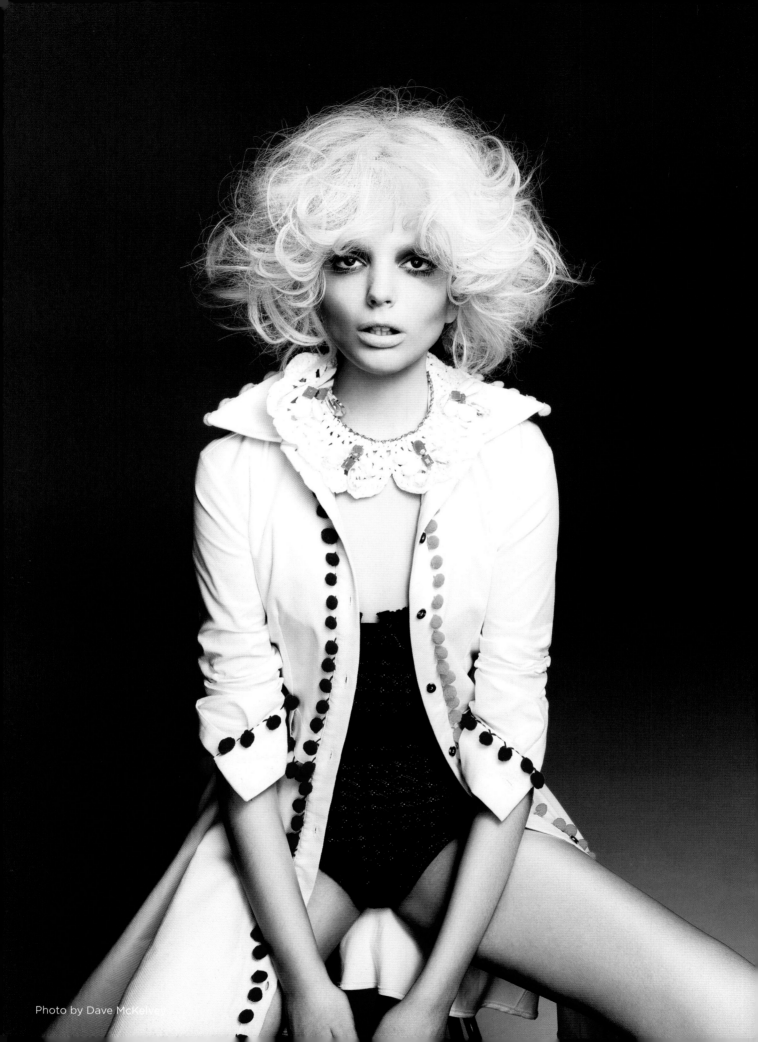

The best colour in the world is the one that looks good on you

— COCO CHANEL

Toolkit

As any good tradesperson will tell you, having the right tool for the job is crucial. Good-quality brushes are vital for blending everything — and the key to flawless makeup is all in the blending. Makeup glides on more easily with a brush — and it stays on.

As a makeup artist, I've collected an abundance of brushes, tweezers and lash curlers over the years, but you only need a few well-chosen essentials to get started. There's a vast array of brushes available, but your starter-kit must-haves should include a long-haired eye blending brush, a short-haired shadow brush, a pointer brush, a blush brush, a brow brush and a contour brush. Look after your brushes and they will last a lifetime. Wash natural-hair brushes once a week with shampoo to keep them clean and lie them flat to dry. (This stops the wooden handles rotting.) Use laundry stain stick for synthetic brushes.

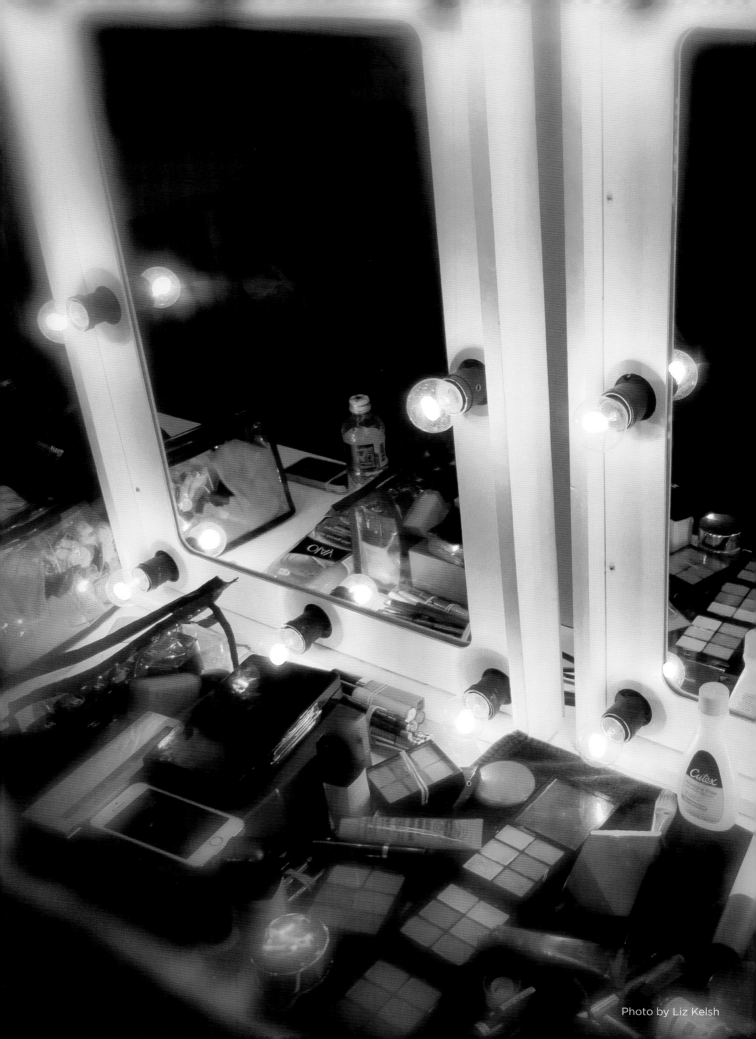

Brush up on basics

Brushes come in synthetic and natural-hair types. Natural-hair brushes, which may be made from goat, sable or squirrel, are well worth the investment and make blending blush and eyeshadow a breeze. Synthetic brushes are best for applying concealer, foundation and lipstick.

Natural-hair brush arsenal

- **LONG-HAIRED EYE BLENDING BRUSH** Must have: this is an absolute essential and should be your first purchase; it will change your life. It's great for seamlessly blending coloured eyeshadows and fading out the edges.

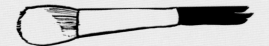

- **SHORT-HAIRED SHADOW BRUSH** Great for applying precision eyeshadow to the crease of the eye.

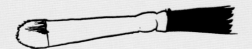

- **SMALL SHORT-HAIRED SHADOW BRUSH** For even greater precision.

- **SHORT-HAIRED POINTER BRUSH** Great for applying shadow to finer areas such as under the eye or along the lashline.

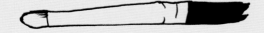

- **LONG-HAIRED POINTER BRUSH** This brush is amazing for blending shadow on the lower lashline.
- **SLANT BRUSH** Good for filling in brows or applying eyeliner.
- **LARGE POWDER BRUSH** As the name suggests, use this brush for applying powder and bronzer.

- **BLUSH BRUSH** A must-have for correct placement of powder blush.

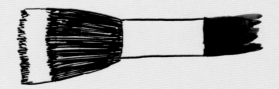

- **CONTOUR BRUSH** Makes contouring a breeze.

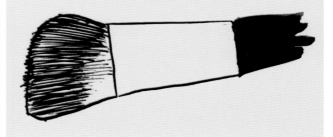

Synthetic brushes

- **SMALL FIBRE-OPTIC BRUSH** Ideal for cream blush and foundation application.
- **LARGE FIBRE-OPTIC BRUSH** This brush is great for foundation, cream bronzer and for powder foundation with a sheer coverage.
- **FOUNDATION BRUSH** Great for applying liquid and cream foundation.
- **LIP BRUSH** This little beauty will have your lipstick perfectly placed. It cuts down wastage too because you use less product than if you apply it straight from the bullet.

- **BROW BRUSH** Essential for subtly feathering brow powder to brows.

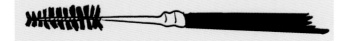

- **CONCEALER BRUSH** Similar to a lip brush but slightly larger, this is great for precise application of concealer.

Add to cart

These essential tools should make an appearance in every makeup kit:

- **SLANT TWEEZERS** You can't live without these. They're great for tweezing stray brow hairs and applying individual false lashes.
- **STRIP LASH APPLICATION TWEEZERS** Makes applying strip lashes less finicky.
- **EYELASH GLUE** For adhering individual and strip lashes.
- **PENCIL SHARPENER** Keeping eye pencils sharp and clean leads to precision application.
- **LASH CURLERS** Always curl your lashes with a regular curler before applying mascara — it opens up the eye area. Use a heated lash curler for quicker results.
- **POWDER PUFF** Using a puff helps press loose powder into foundation, making it last longer.
- **THE HUMBLE COTTON BUD** Where would we be without the cotton bud? I always have these on hand to clean up any makeup mishaps or mistakes.

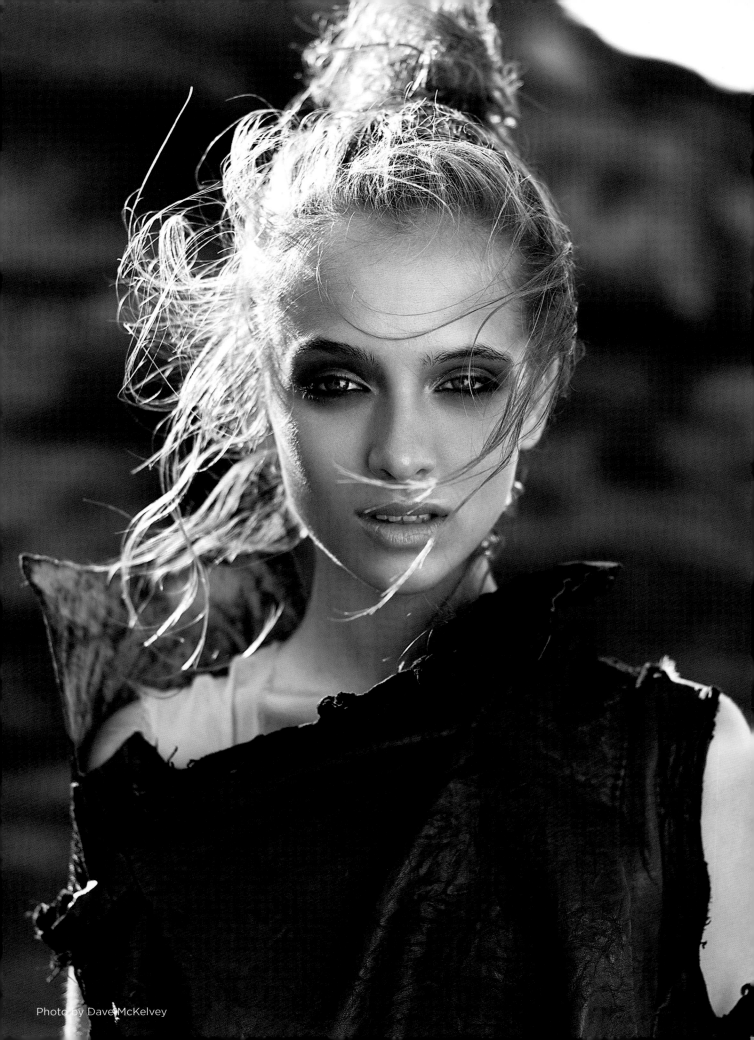

Cosmetic wardrobe

Now let's look at what you'll need in your basic makeup kit. For starters, you must have two or three bases. Try a BB cream for weekend wear — it will give you a light coverage, along with the all-important SPF protection. Use a cream foundation and concealer during the week for fuller coverage and a translucent powder compact for touch-ups on the go. To get the facial palette looking flawless, finish with an artfully placed cream highlighter.

A collection of neutral eyeshadows is compulsory, ranging from taupe to brown to black, with a couple of metallic options — including a silver and bronze — thrown in for good measure. A taupe cream eyeshadow is an essential base for most looks or it can be worn on its own.

Pencil liners — a black and a brown — to define eyes are also a must in the beauty arsenal, coupled with a thickening and lengthening mascara in black.

For cheeks, a coral-based cream blush — as well as a pink one — will create a natural blushing glow.

And the five must-haves for lips are a soft natural nude lipstick and matching lipliner; a classic red lipstick and matching lipliner; and a nude lip gloss.

A brow kit is a great investment. It includes powder and a pencil to create perfectly defined brows.

Tip

To avoid a makeup rut, invest in two new items each season.

Face

The rules of foundation

Finding the perfect foundation match for your skin is makeup's holy grail. With so many foundation choices around, where do you begin? The search stops here. I'll give you the knowledge to choose the best foundation every time.

There are three main considerations when selecting a foundation: texture, coverage and colour.

Tip

Spend a few minutes massaging moisturiser into the face before applying foundation. Your skin will glow and the foundation will last longer.

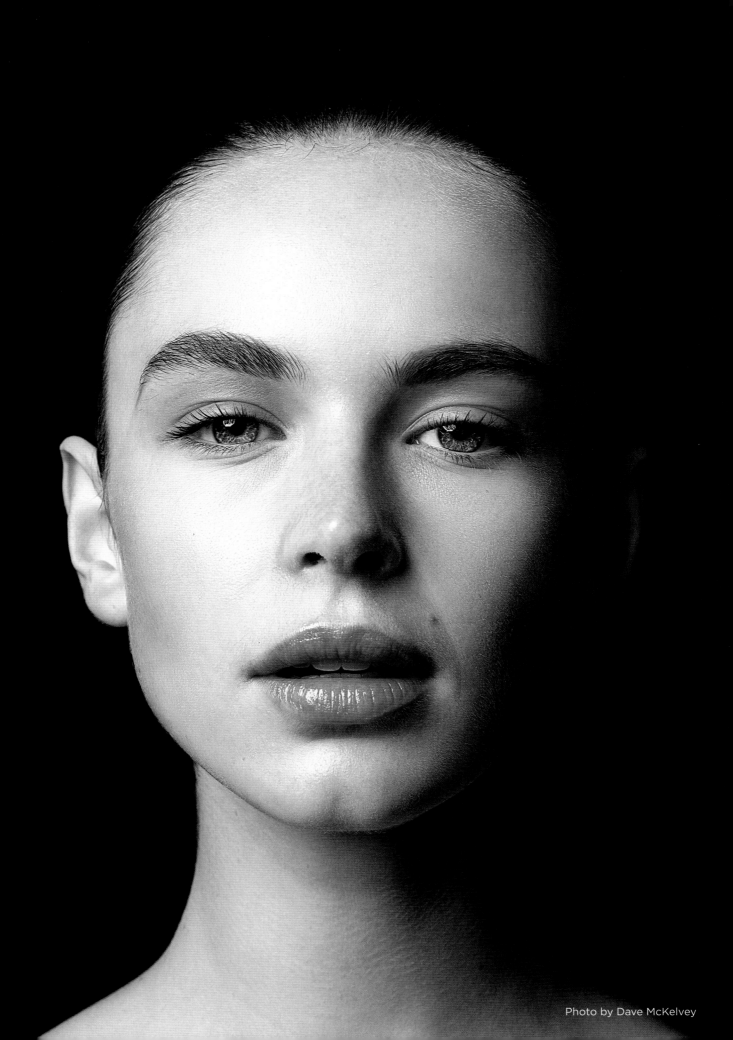

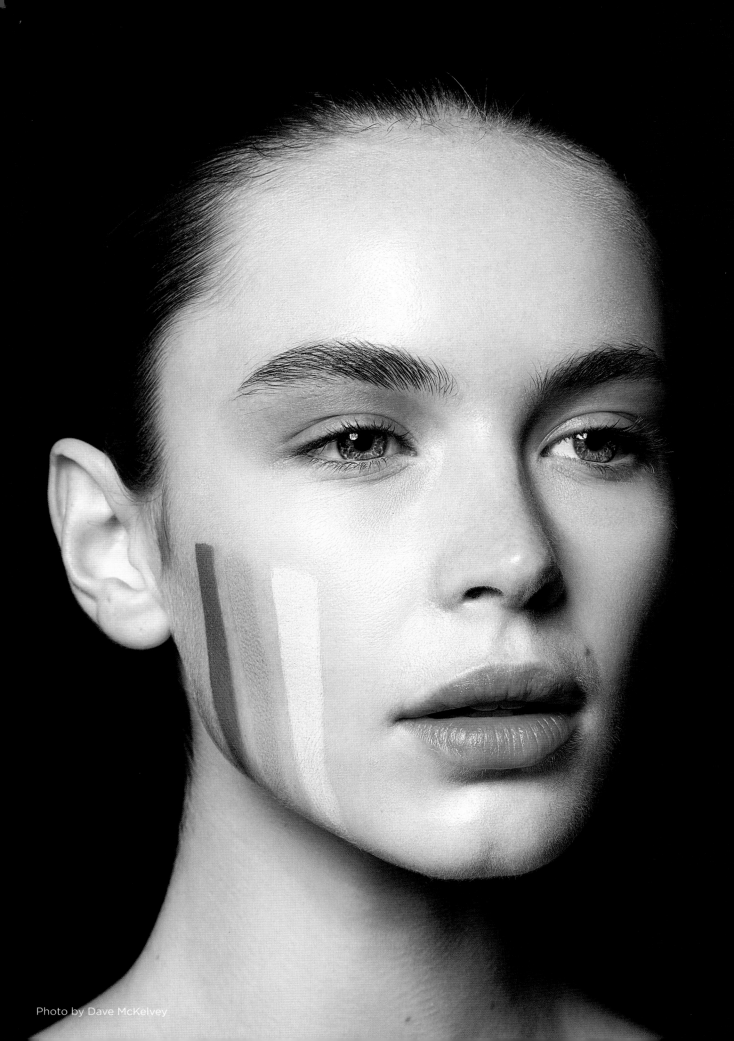

Photo by Dave McKelvey

Texture

What type of finish are you?

- **DEWY** — generally preferred by those with dry skin.
- **MATT** — great if you have oily skin or if you tend to get lots of shine. My preference is an oil-free matt foundation.
- **SATIN** — my personal favourite, sitting somewhere between dewy and matt. This is my favourite 'red-carpet' finish.

Coverage

Sheer, medium or full?

- **SHEER OR LIGHT FINISH** — a transparent foundation for those with relatively clear skin that needs just a little coverage. This type of foundation gives the most natural finish.
- **MEDIUM** — less transparent than sheer but it will cover most skin imperfections such as redness or light pigmentation. This is my favourite because it also looks natural.
- **FULL** — totally covers the skin with no transparency. It covers a multitude of sins but can have a very heavy appearance.

Colour

Although there are pink-based and yellow-based foundations, I generally prefer yellow-based foundations as they tend to suit most skin types. Pink-based foundations can look a little grey and are most suited to the fairest of fair skins.

Make a rough guess at the shade you think may suit you and then choose three shades close to that. Apply one stripe of each colour along the jawline and onto the neck. The correct shade will be the one that practically disappears into the skin. Store lighting can be challenging, so carry a compact mirror and walk into natural daylight to check your choice prior to purchasing.

What's out there

TINTED MOISTURISER AND BB CREAM

These are sheer, with minimal coverage and a soft dewy finish. They're great for those who don't like wearing foundation and just want to dip their toe in. They are best applied using the fingers.

LIQUID FOUNDATION

This comes in sheer or medium coverage, all finishes and is easy to apply and blend. It's great for those who tend to have drier skin and is best applied with a foundation brush and then finished with fingers.

MOUSSE FOUNDATION

This may be sheer to medium coverage in a satin to matt finish. This is ideal for those who like their foundation to feel light on the skin. Apply with a brush or sponge to get an even finish.

CREAM FOUNDATION

This is my personal favourite. It creates medium to full coverage with a dewy to satin finish and a luxurious touch. Apply with a brush and fingers or a sponge.

STICK FOUNDATION

Stick foundation creates medium to full coverage and is available in satin to matt finishes. It's best for those who want a fuller foundation and should be applied with a brush or sponge.

POWDER FOUNDATION

Powder foundation has come a long way, especially with the advent of mineral powder foundations. It can be applied directly to the skin and is wonderful for those who like a matt finish with little fuss. It's best applied with a sponge or brush.

POWDER

- Translucent loose powder is used to set and mattify foundation without adding extra colour or coverage. It also helps increase the longevity of the coverage.
- Pressed translucent powder is a fantastic portable touch-up essential.
- Loose powder is pigmented and used to set and mattify foundation by adding a little more coverage.

CONCEALER

In addition to your foundation, everyone should have two concealers — one that's slightly lighter than their foundation and one that matches and blends well, disappearing into their foundation.

PRIMER

Primers are designed to go under foundation and can be useful to make your foundation last longer. But I always think that if you're on the right track with your skincare and you've got the right foundation that works for your skin, then you shouldn't need a primer.

LUMINIZER

A light, reflective cream that can be added to foundation for extra glow or used as a highlighter.

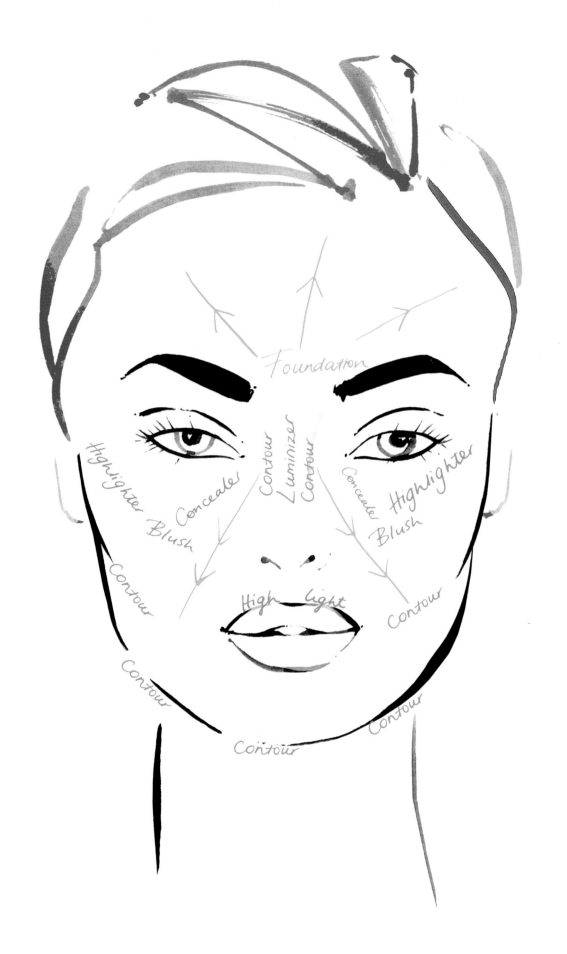

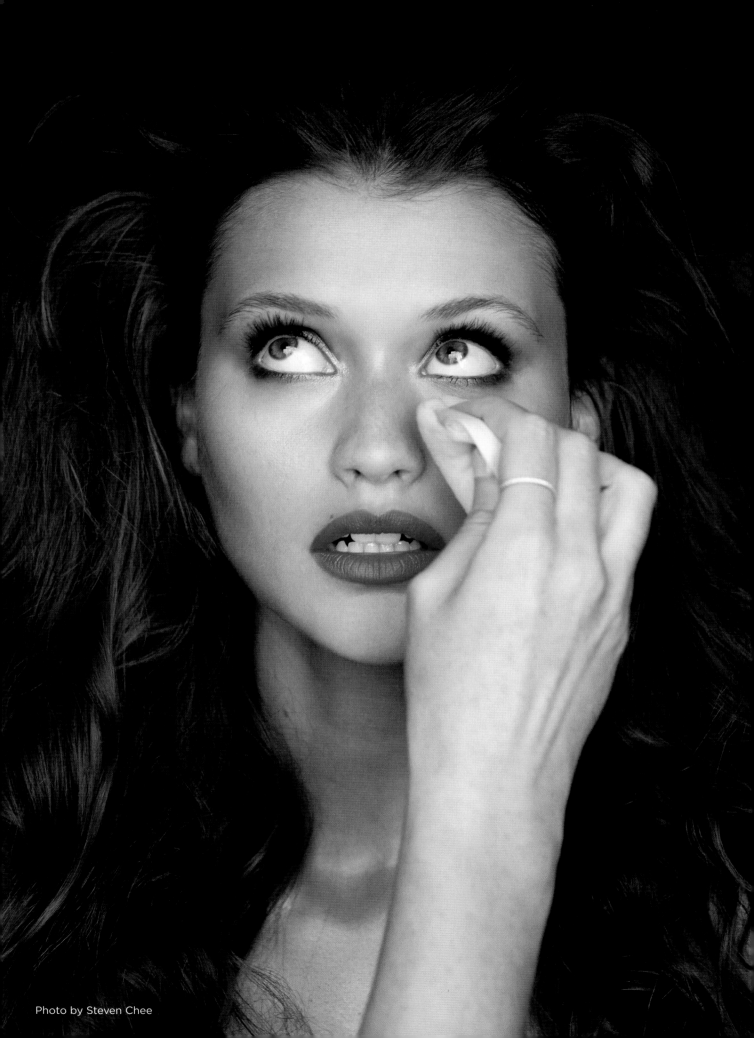

All in the application

1. Cleanse the face to remove any excess oil.
2. Apply moisturiser and spend a few minutes to work it well into the skin. This step is crucial in creating the perfect base because the massaging action ensures the skin is well primed.
3. Apply a primer, if needed, in the centre of your face at the T-zone.
4. Using a foundation brush, your fingers or a sponge, start working the foundation outwards to the hairline. Apply sparingly — it's always easier to add more than it is to take it off. Personally, I prefer to apply with a brush then pat the rest in with my fingers — the warmth of the fingertips helps blend the foundation.
5. Dab on concealer where needed, remembering that under-eye concealer will be slightly lighter than your foundation and concealer for blemishes, pigmentation or areas that need a little help should match your foundation.
6. Apply your powder using a powder puff, lightly pressing and rolling the powder puff onto the face. Concentrate mostly on the T-zone to keep oil at bay.

Tips

Apply concealer where needed after foundation, rather than before. This avoids the cover provided by the concealer from being diluted by the foundation.

If your skin is very oily but you want to keep up with the luminous skin trend, wear matt foundation with a powder highlighter for a radiant, non-greasy look.

Troubleshooting

- If you suffer from breakouts, choose a sheer foundation all over the face and apply concealer where needed.
- Accidently applied too much foundation and feel like you're wearing a mask? Tissue off the excess, rub moisturiser into the palm of your hand and pat onto the skin — it helps 'sheer out' the foundation, making it more translucent.
- If you've applied too much powder and the finished look is a little too cakey, spritz the face with Evian spray to lighten the effect.
- When applying under-eye concealer to dark circles, lower the chin and look in the mirror — this will make the dark circles pop out. Now, with a fine concealer brush, apply concealer only to the dark area on the inner corner of the eye and blend.
- Be very light-handed when applying foundation, powder or concealer to the outer corner of the eye — too heavy an application can lead to creasing. If you've applied too much to this area and it looks creased, just dab a little eye cream on top to blend it out.
- Remember — your perfect colour match may be a combination of two foundations mixed together. Your skin can vary its shade with the changing seasons too so it's always good to have a lighter and slightly darker foundation to blend together. Think of it as customising your perfect foundation shade.

Tip

Have you ever seen a photo of yourself where your face seems white and your neck looks tan? That's because the foundation and powder on your face reflects light and the skin on your neck absorbs it, making it look darker (known as ghosting). If you're going to an event where you're likely to be snapped, avoid this effect by dusting a little translucent powder on your neck and décolletage.

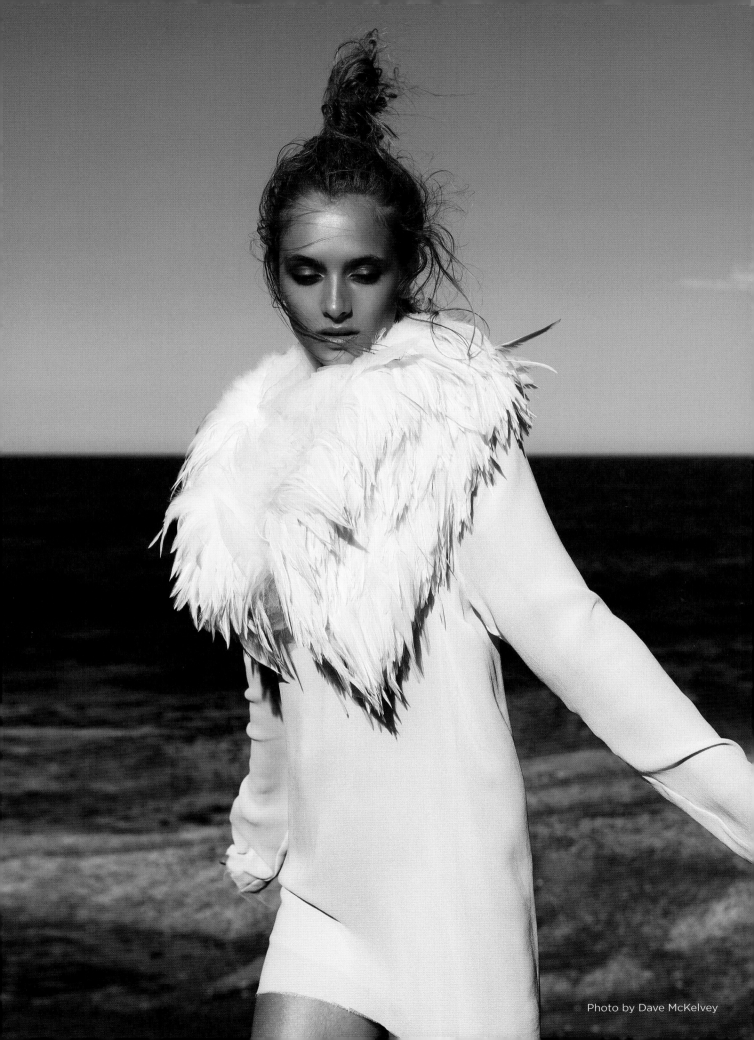

Photo by Dave McKelvey

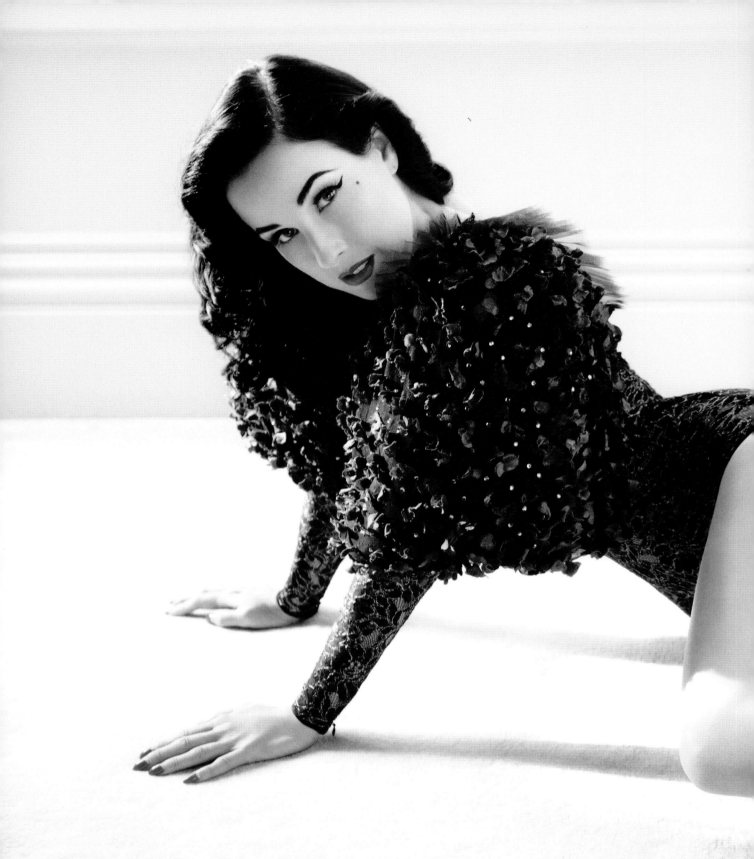

Photo by Simon Lekias

I love glamour and artificial beauty. I love the idea of artifice and dressing up and makeup and hair

— *DITA VON TEESE*

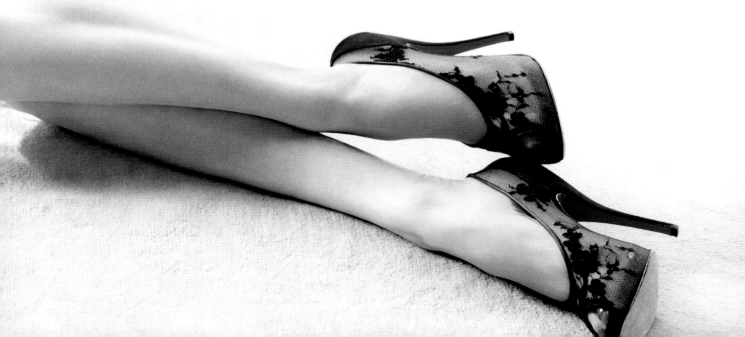

The art of contouring and highlighting

The ability to work with light and shading is the backbone of makeup illusion. I'm obsessed with highlighting and contouring and, even after 20 years in the industry, I still find myself constantly amazed at how this wizardly technique can transform a face.

It works like this: darker or matt products absorb light, creating a shadow or giving the illusion of something receding. This technique helps to conceal a double chin, for instance. Light or shimmery products reflect light, giving an illusion of prominence, so this can be used to make, say, cheekbones appear more eye-catching.

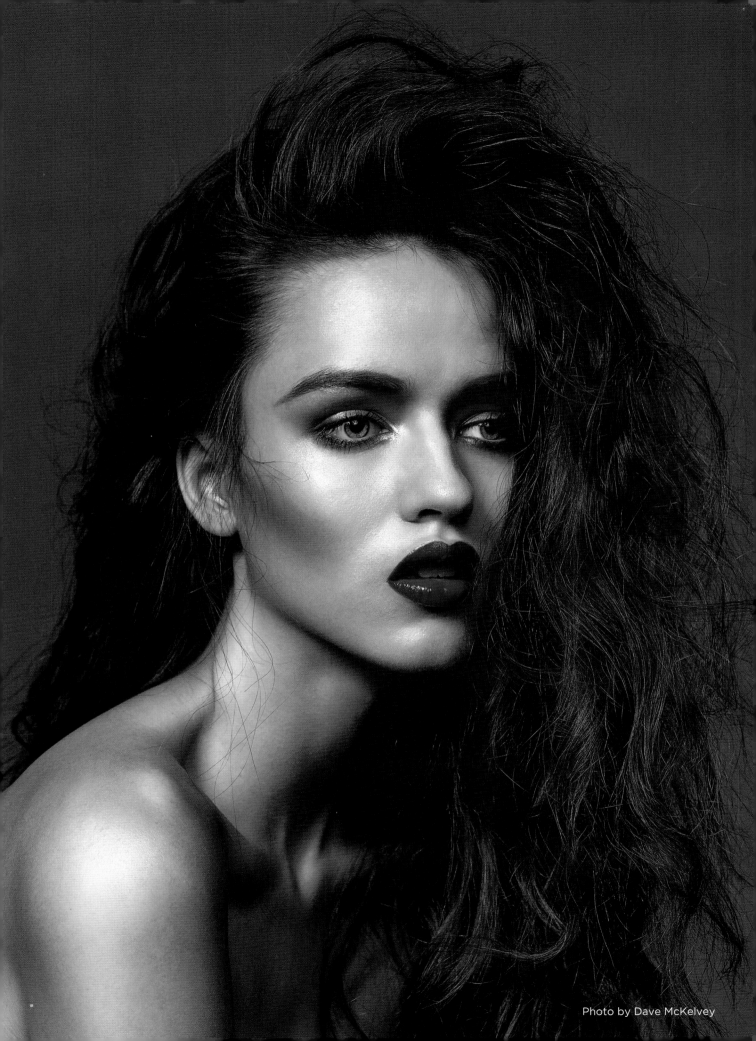

Photo by Dave McKelvey

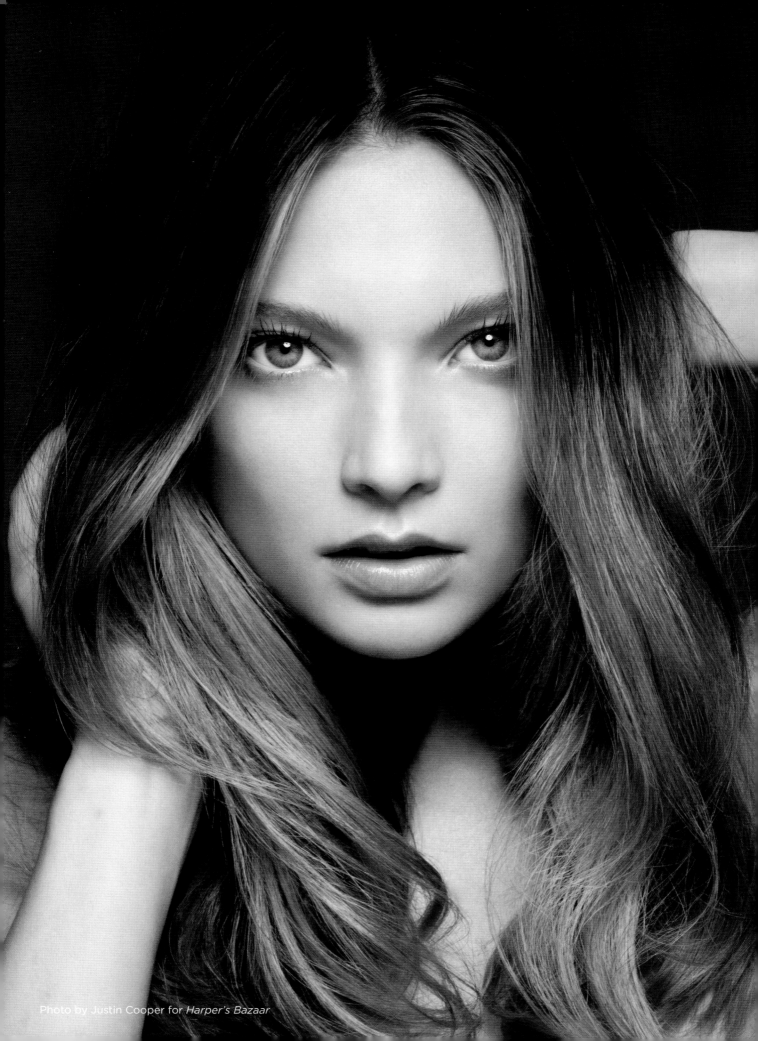

Why contour? Let me count the ways

- To create stronger cheekbones.
- To narrow the nose.
- To define the jawline.
- To minimise a large forehead.

What you'll need

First up, a cream or powder contouring product can be applied with a sponge or a brush — personally, I prefer a brush. It should be matt in consistency and a taupe-coloured powder or cream, or a darker-coloured foundation.

Before you begin, imagine a skull, thinking about where the natural hollows occur. Observe your face in the mirror, turning slowly from side to side, noting where the light naturally reflects from the skin. Now, we're going to give nature a little boost to help accentuate the bone structure using highlighting and contouring. When contouring, it's vital to make sure the product is well blended.

CHEEKS

First, suck in your cheeks to create a 'fish face'. Using a contouring brush, apply the product *sparingly* to the hollows of the cheeks. (The position will vary from face to face, depending on your natural hollows.) Now, relax your cheeks and blend the edges to create the contoured effect.

JAWLINE

Apply contouring product just below the jawline, starting under the ear. (Personally, I wouldn't be seen dead without a little contour just under my chin!)

FOREHEAD

A little contouring product on the temples looks great on most faces. If you have a large forehead, apply some shading all along the hairline of the forehead. And make sure to blend, blend, blend.

NOSE

A little shading along each side of a wide nose works wonders. To make a bulbous nose appear smaller, apply a touch of shading on each side of the tip.

Tip

Don't use shimmer bronzer to contour, as the shimmer reflects too much light and contouring is all about creating shadow.

Why highlight?
Why not!

- To bring out cheekbones.
- To narrow the nose.
- To add dimension to a flat face.
- To add length to a short face.

What you'll need

A highlighter may be a lighter-coloured foundation, a highlighting powder, or a natural-toned shimmer powder or cream, and can be applied with a brush or a sponge.

Highlighter is applied to areas of the face that you want to be more prominent.

CHEEKS
A touch of highlighter placed on the top of the cheekbones is a must, day or night.

NOSE
A little highlighter applied down the centre of the nose can narrow it, but also adds a flattering glow to makeup.

CHIN AND FOREHEAD
Applying matt highlighter to the centre of the forehead between the brows and also on the centre of the chin helps elongate the face.

Troubleshooting

- Don't use a shimmer product to contour.
- Apply products precisely and then blend subtly for best results. The aim is to create definition to the face without severe lines.
- Less is definitely more when it comes to highlighting and contouring.
- Always apply highlighting and contouring in good light, to avoid any nasty surprises.

Tip

Dab a little highlighter on the cheekbones to add definition and radiance.

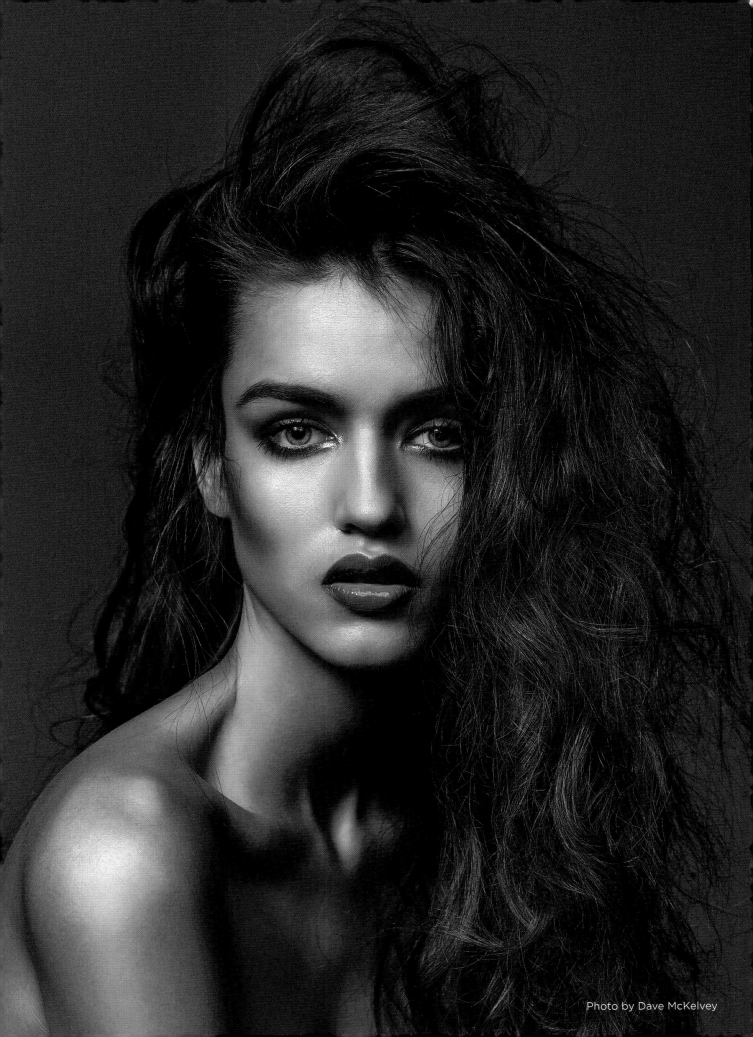

Photo by Dave McKelvey

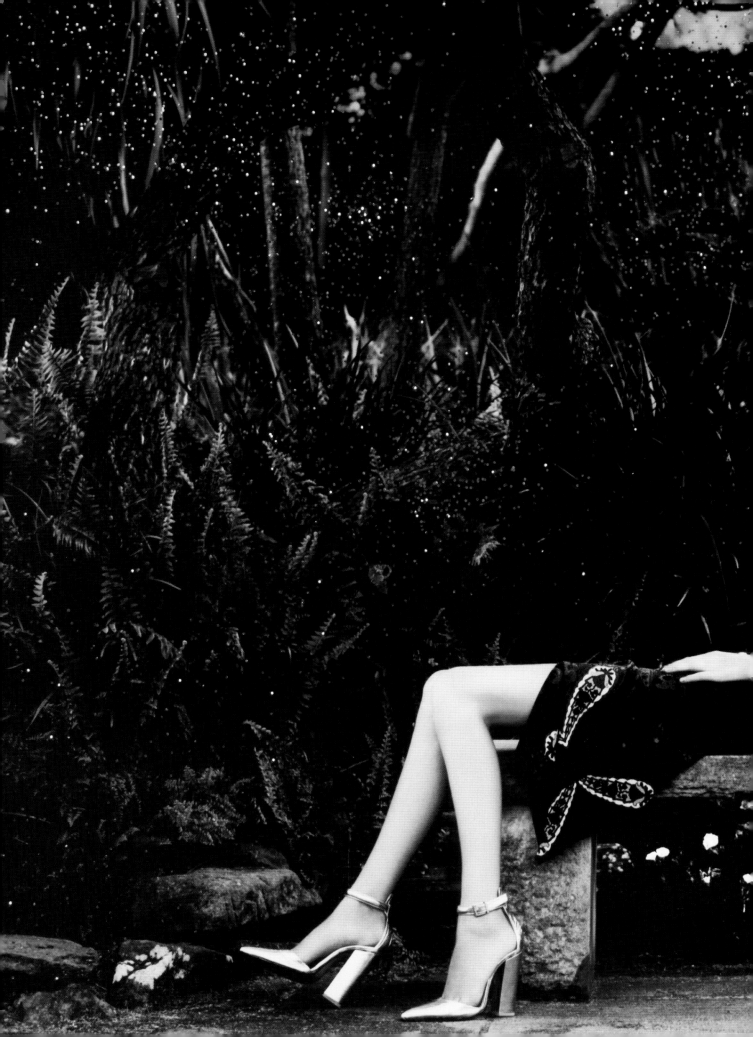

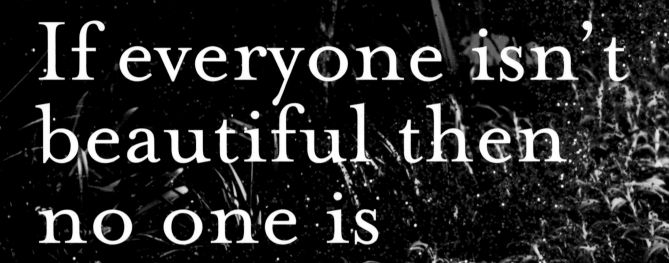

If everyone isn't beautiful then no one is

— ANDY WARHOL

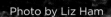

Blushed
for success

OK, let's start with a very simple statement: blush and bronzer are two entirely different things. They are as different as mascara and lipstick and both have their functions to perform. And yes, you can wear blush and bronzer at the same time! Bronzer comes in various shades of tan and is designed to give the skin a sun-kissed look; blush comes in tones of pink and orange and gives you a healthy flush. Blush breathes life back into a tired, lacklustre face and provides an instant pick-me-up. It can be the mainstay of an almost natural look as well as adding balance to sultry smoky eyes.

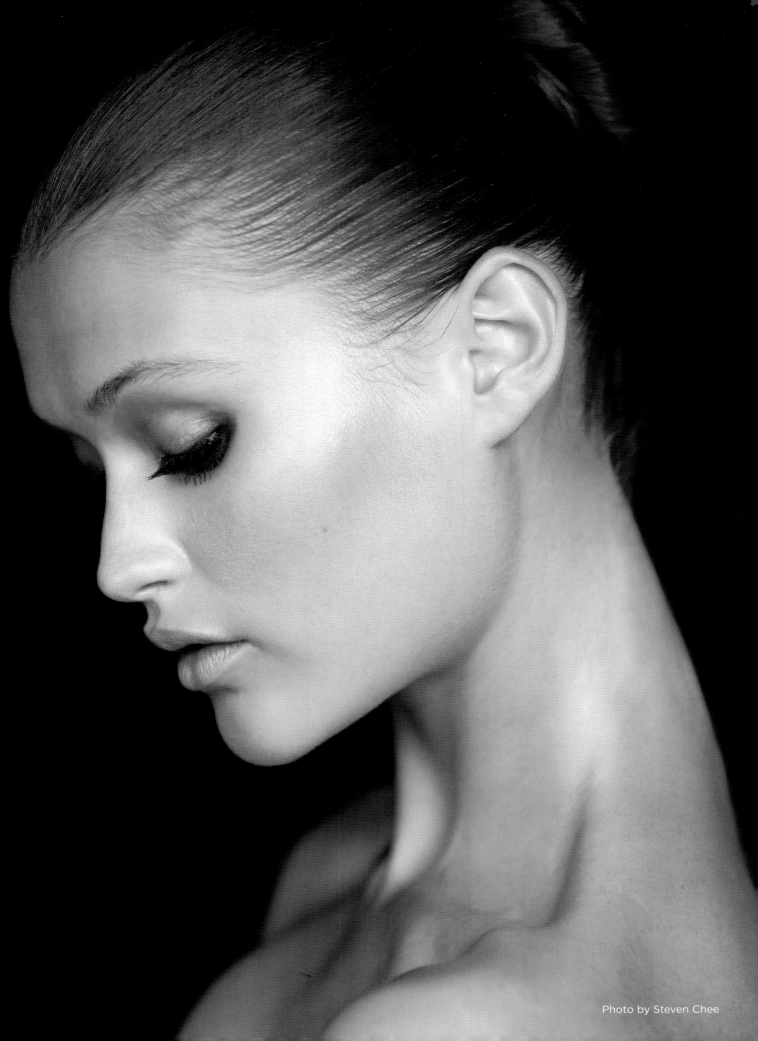

Photo by Steven Chee

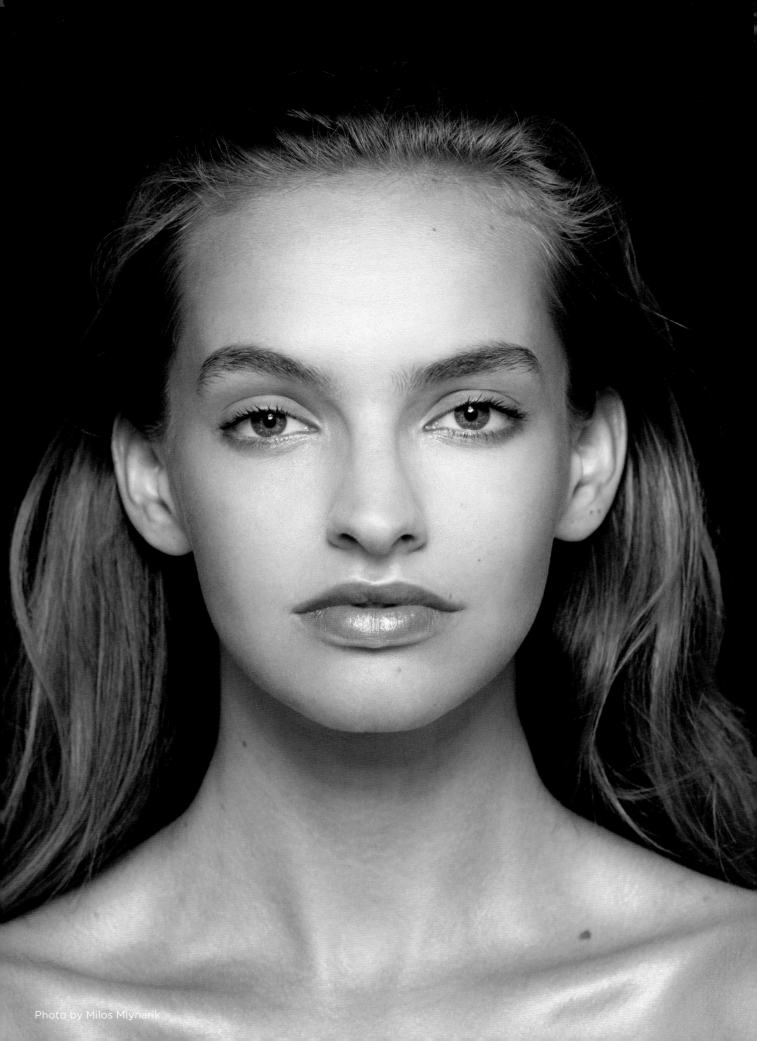

Photo by Milos Mlynarik

Blush basics

- **LIQUID** This is great for oily skin and has amazing lasting power. Apply it with a foundation brush over your foundation, or you can apply to nude skin (no foundation base, just moisturiser).
- **GEL TINTS** These are a great two-in-one because they can also be applied to lips, adding just a kiss of colour. Gel tints have long staying power and are wonderful for most skin types. Apply with fingers and blend with a brush.
- **CREAM** Particularly good for dry skin, cream blush looks good on everyone. Apply with fingers and blend. It has medium staying power and illuminates the face.
- **MATT POWDER** Long-lasting and perfect for problem skin, matt powder must be worn over foundation and powder and applied with a blush brush.
- **SHIMMER POWDER** This gives the glow of a cream with the lasting power of a powder. It's not ideal for problem skin and should be worn over foundation and powder. Apply with a blush brush.

Now you're familiar with the categories, let's talk shades. Pink and berry hues give a healthy, flushed look, while orange, coral and peach tones add warmth and depth to the face. You can wear either hue, although sticking to your skin tone will look more natural, and choosing the opposite tone will pop more.

The most important thing to remember is match your blush tone to your lip colour — for example, pink lips go with pink blush and for blue-based red lipstick use pink or berry-toned blush. Orange-toned blush works best with orange-based red lipstick.

To apply blush correctly, look into the mirror and smile. Locate the 'apples' of the cheeks and apply a small amount of blush to this area. Stop smiling and blend the blush upward and outward towards the hairline.

Tip

Cleanse your face twice before bed — the first time removes makeup and the second cleanses the skin.

On the model opposite, I used a cream blusher for both her lips and her cheeks. Liquids, gel tints and creams are all great multi-use products.

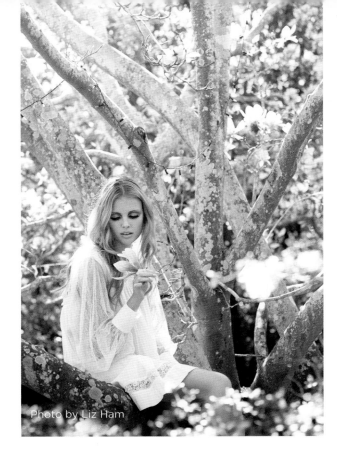

Photo by Liz Ham

Troubleshooting

- Always keep blush and lips a similar tone — mismatches make for 'ruddy' makeup.
- Don't be afraid to mix blush colours together: if one is too vibrant and the other is too light, mix them together for a whole new colour.
- Less is more. Always apply blush sparingly because it's much easier to build up colour than it is to knock it back.

- Gel, liquid and cream blush are great on bare skin or liquid foundation.
- Powder blush works better on a powdered base. Stick to this rule and you should have no problem blending.
- With problem skin, your best bet is a matt base with a matt powder blush.

Tip

If you have very reactive skin, try splashing it with sparkling mineral water. It really calms skin down while closing the pores.

On the model opposite, I've created a soft coral lip and reflected that in the blush for a subtle yet beautiful look.

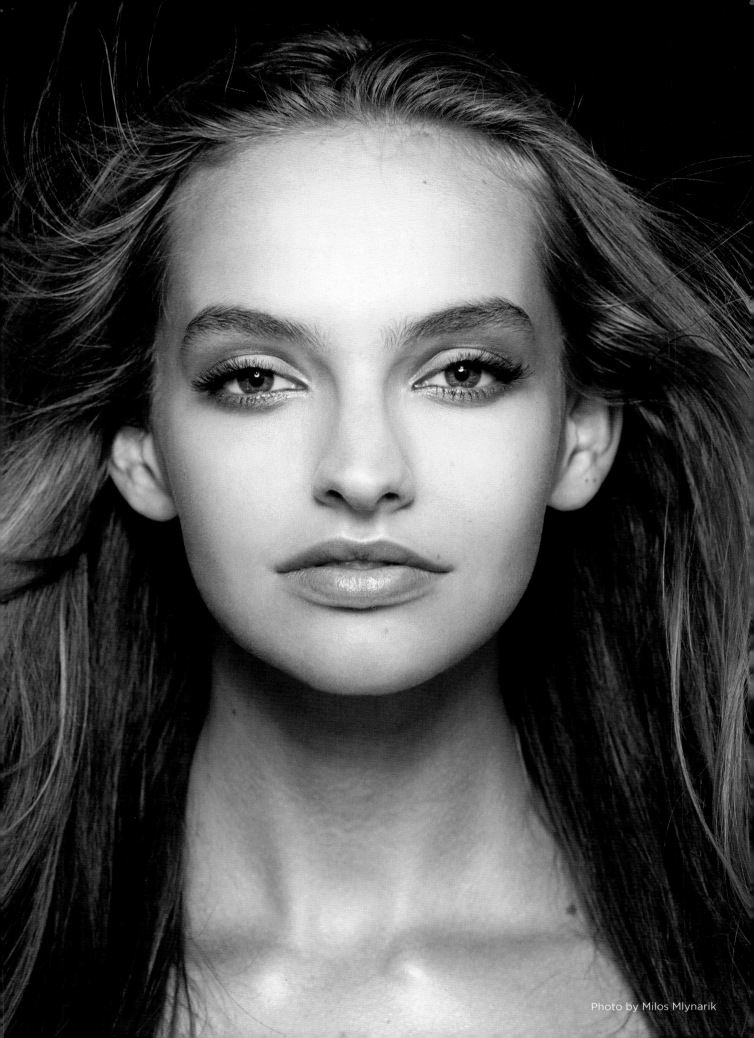

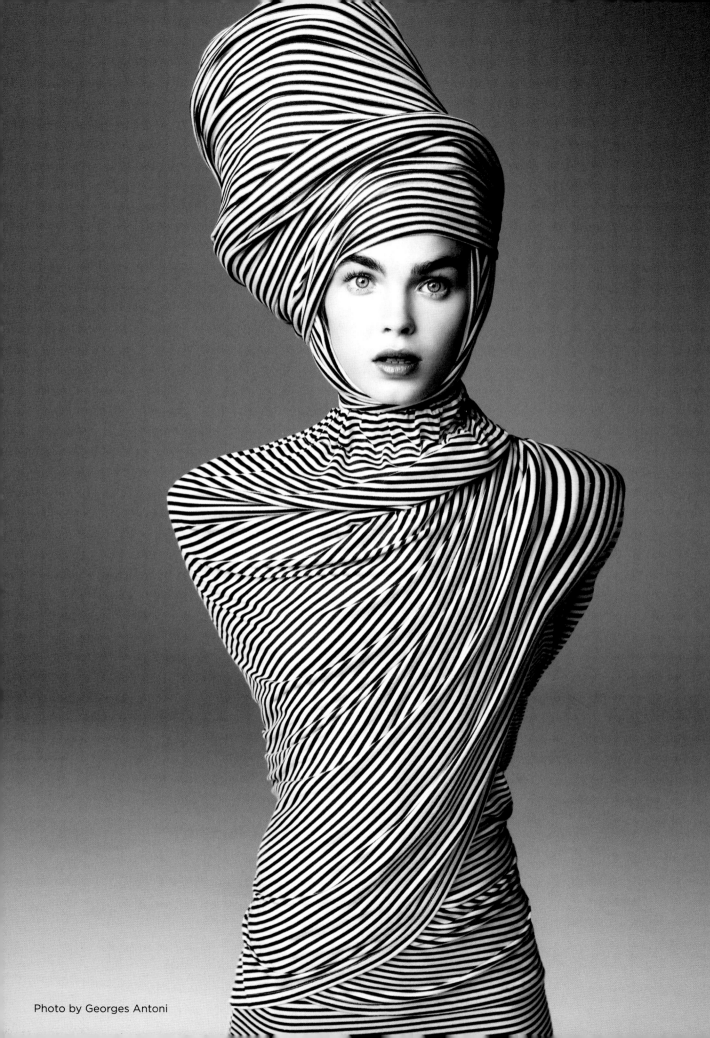

When asked by his Careers Officer, 'What can you do better than others?' Boy George replied, 'Makeup'

Bronzed
and beautiful

Bronzer is your new best friend. Strategically placed, it can give your face a healthy glow. The first thing I do when I'm feeling a little tired is add a touch more bronzer — it gives my face radiance. As an added bonus, people then say how good I look, helping me forget how tired I actually am and that I started my day at 4 a.m.

A word of warning, however: bronzer is only ever meant to be a subtle glow. Use it sparingly for best results. As a rule, fair skin tones suit peach-based bronzers, while medium-toned skin looks best with a honey tint. Darker skin benefits from a warm, brick-based colour.

Tip
Always apply bronzer with a large brush.

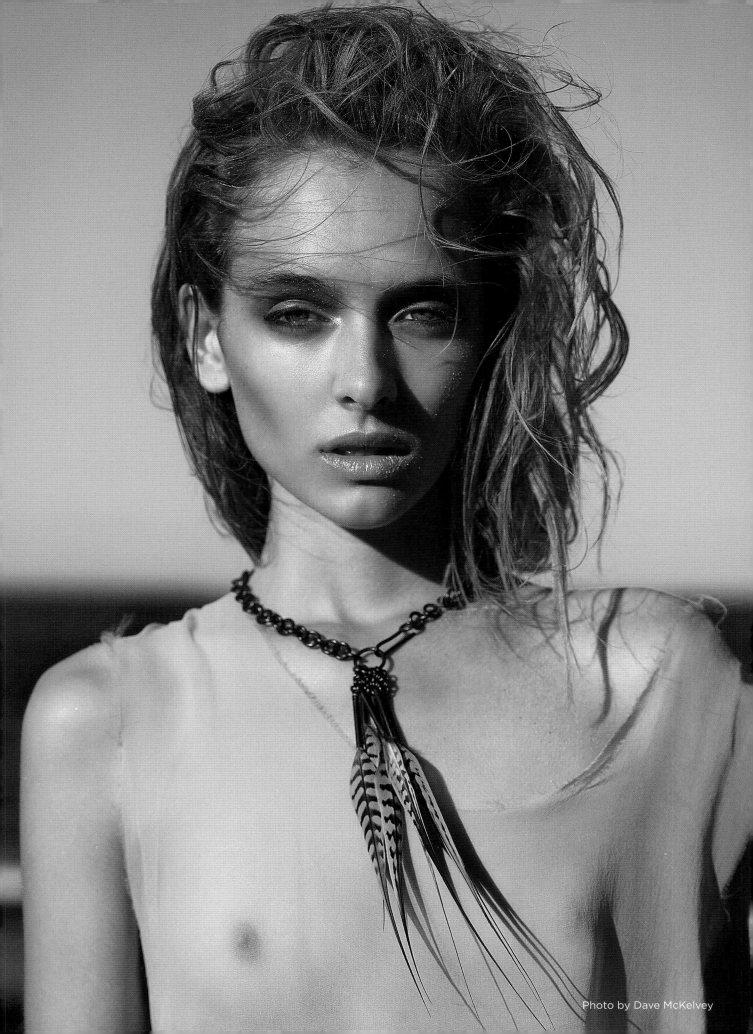

Photo by Dave McKelvey

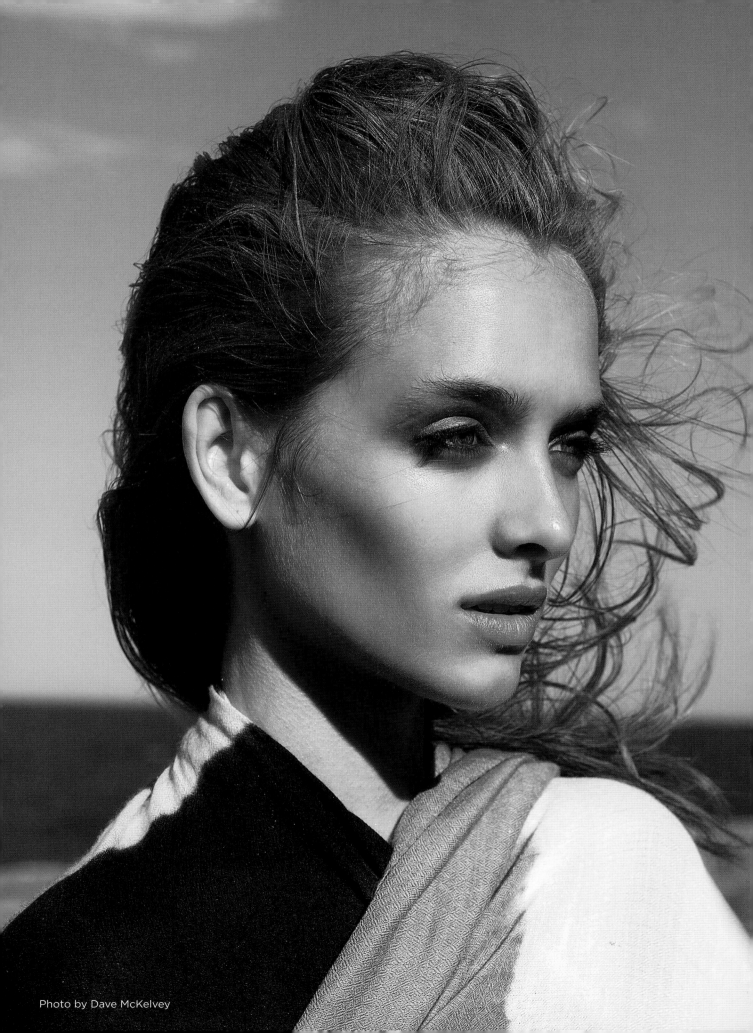

The bronzing wardrobe

- **LIQUID** This bronzer is long-lasting, usually waterproof (great for the beach) and is best worn on bare skin. Apply with a foundation brush and then blend with a fibre-optic brush or a makeup sponge. Note: don't apply it over foundation or powder.
- **GEL** This formula lasts well and can be worn on bare skin, creating a very natural finish. Again, it's a great option for the beach or a no-makeup day — because we all know there is no such thing as an absolutely no-makeup day.
- **CREAM** This is my favourite because it suits all skin types and can be worn on bare skin or over foundation. Apply with a large brush.
- **MATT POWDER** Don't go there if your skin is dry but this is a great choice for problem skin. It works best over foundation and/or powder. At a pinch, it can be worn on bare skin but it will take a bit of blending. Apply with a big bronzing brush.
- **SHIMMER POWDER** This powder is not a great option for problem skin but works well for dry skin as the shimmer gives the illusion of hydration. Be aware that the added shimmer in this bronzer will make it more obvious to the eye, so go lightly. Apply with a large bronzing brush.

When applying bronzer, think about where your face naturally catches the sun because this is where you want to apply it: basically, cheeks, forehead and chin. Using a large bronzing brush, start applying it to the perimeter of the face in big circular motions, then finish with a light dusting across the nose and chin.

Troubleshooting

- Remember, the key to cream and powder bronzers is using a large brush.
- If you feel you've overdone it, spray the face with a little Evian spray and blend more with a brush.
- Don't forget to blend down onto the neck and décolletage and finish with a light dusting on the backs of the hands.

Tip

Invest in a good eye cream. The skin around the eyes is more delicate and regular face cream is too heavy.

Lips
— a lip service

Lipstick can make or break a look. It's the quickest way to add the 'wow' factor to your makeup every time. The right colour and correct application can accessorise and revitalise a plain outfit. Beautiful lipstick can even add sparkle to an otherwise dull day.

Before you start, consider that no lipstick or gloss looks good on dry, cracked lips. It's a good time to get into the habit of exfoliating with a lip scrub and using a lip balm at night. Just like foundation, the main things you need to consider when choosing a lip product are colour, texture and performance.

Tip

Try mixing it up a bit: change the texture of your lipstick by adding a little clear gloss to a matt lipstick or by dabbing some translucent powder over a satin-finish lipstick.

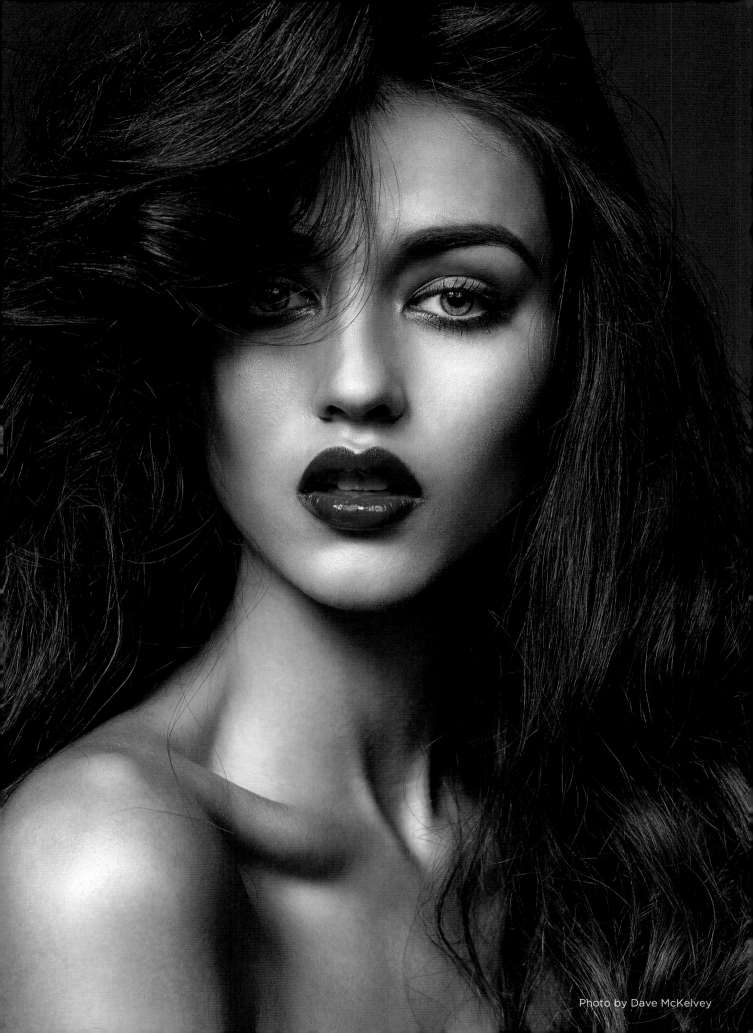

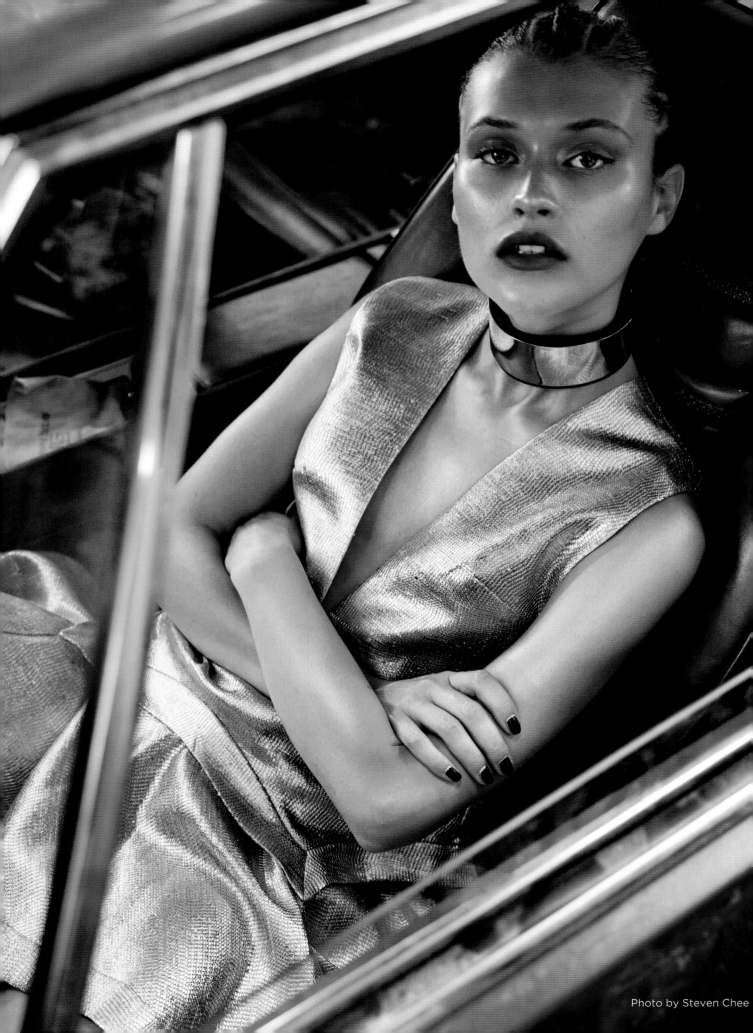

Texture and coverage

Do you want a gloss, satin or matt finish? How transparent do you want the product to be?

- **STAIN** — very easy to wear and a great way to try a strong colour in a subtle way.
- **GLOSS** — easy to apply and can be used with or without lipliner. It gives a sheer glossy finish and will need multiple touchups throughout the day.
- **SHEER LIPSTICK** — similar to gloss, but not as shiny — and a little more long-wearing.
- **CREAM LIPSTICK** — full coverage with a creamy satin finish and easy to wear, particularly in nude colours. It can be used with or without lipliner.
- **MATT LIPSTICK** — full coverage with a matt finish. Great for statement lips and works best when paired with a matching liner.

- **LIP PENS** — these give a stain to the lips and are very long-wearing.
- **LIP CRAYONS** — come in matt and satin finishes and are ideal for on-the-go application.
- **LONG-WEAR LIPSTICK** — sometimes called liquid lipsticks, these are ideal for helping combat lipstick migrating into the liplines.
- **TINTED LIP BALM** — fantastic for the no-makeup look. Adds a touch of colour while moisturising the lips at the same time.
- **MOISTURISING LIPSTICK** — comes in all finishes and is great for those who suffer from dry lips.

Tips

The night before applying 'statement lips', exfoliate and apply a lip conditioner to ensure the perfect pout.

Get double wear from your stronger lip colours by dabbing them on with your finger. The result? A modern lip stain.

The perfect nude

Everyone should have their 'go to' nude. Your perfect nude colour will ideally be just a couple of shades darker than your natural lip colour. When shopping for a new lip colour, try it on without a trace of other makeup. The right colour should instantly bring life to your face; the wrong colour will make you look more washed out.

Liner

When applying liner, always work with your natural lipline and then blend that line with a brush before applying your lipstick.

Tip

Keep lips and blush a similar tone. If you're wearing a pink lipstick, go for a pinkish blush; with coral lips choose a peach blush.

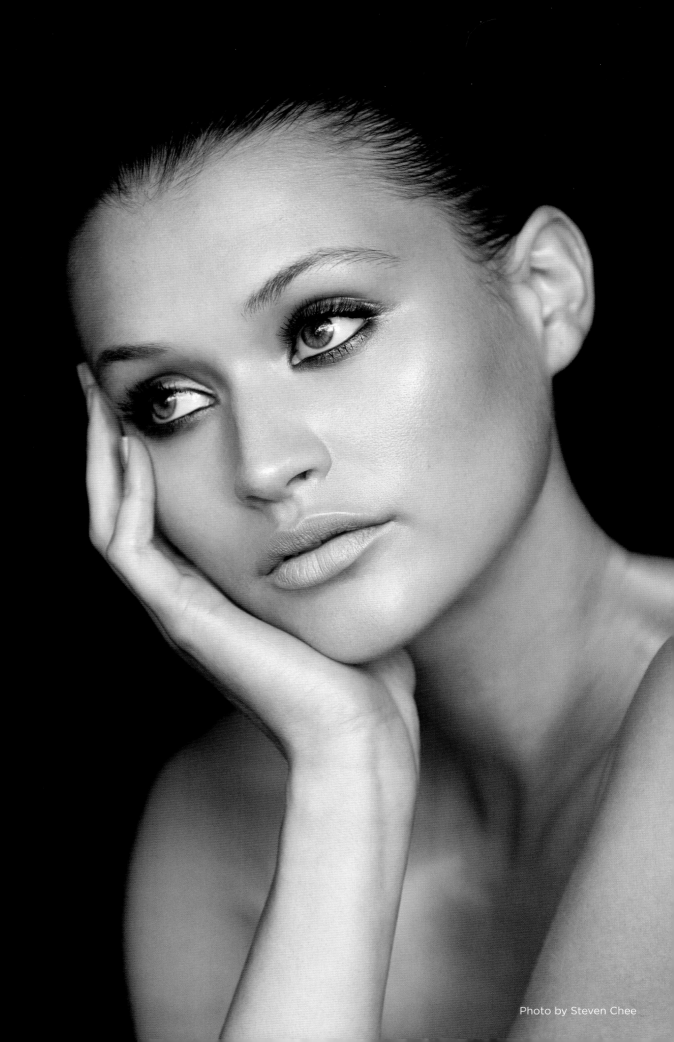

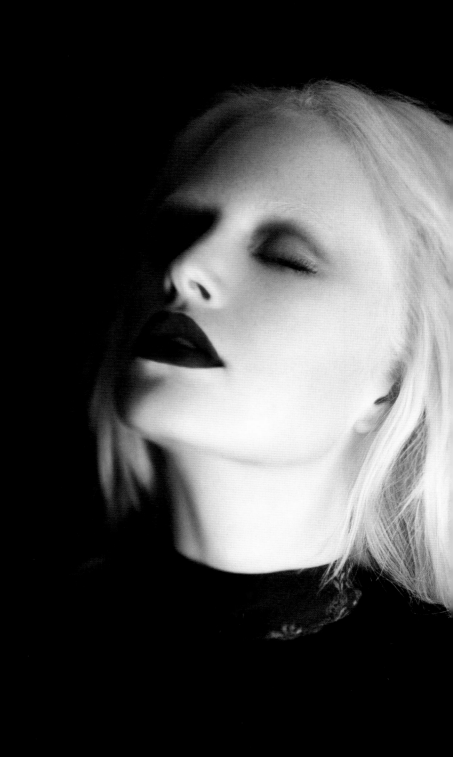

Photo by Liz Ham

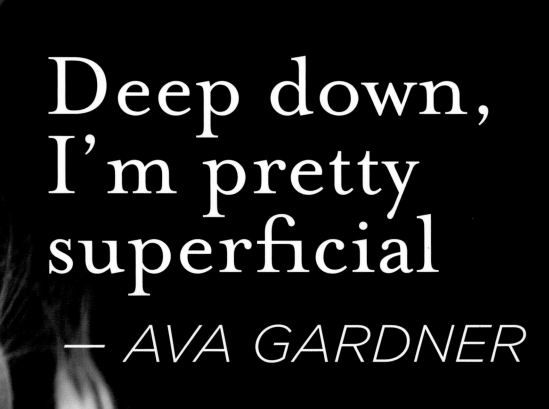

Deep down,
I'm pretty
superficial

— *AVA GARDNER*

Eyes

Brows
— the face-framer

But speak you this with a sad brow?

— WILLIAM SHAKESPEARE, *MUCH ADO ABOUT NOTHING*

The quote says it all, really. Skinny, over-plucked brows can make the whole face appear skeletal. The brow rule clearly states: 'The thinner the brows, the older the look.' By contrast, well-groomed eyebrows are your best facial friend — they add definition to your eyes and jawline, giving an overall frame to your face. The most flattering brow is a skilfully groomed version of your natural brow.

Tip

Well-groomed brows frame the face and give sophistication to every look. To enhance brow shape, choose a pencil slightly lighter than your natural colour.

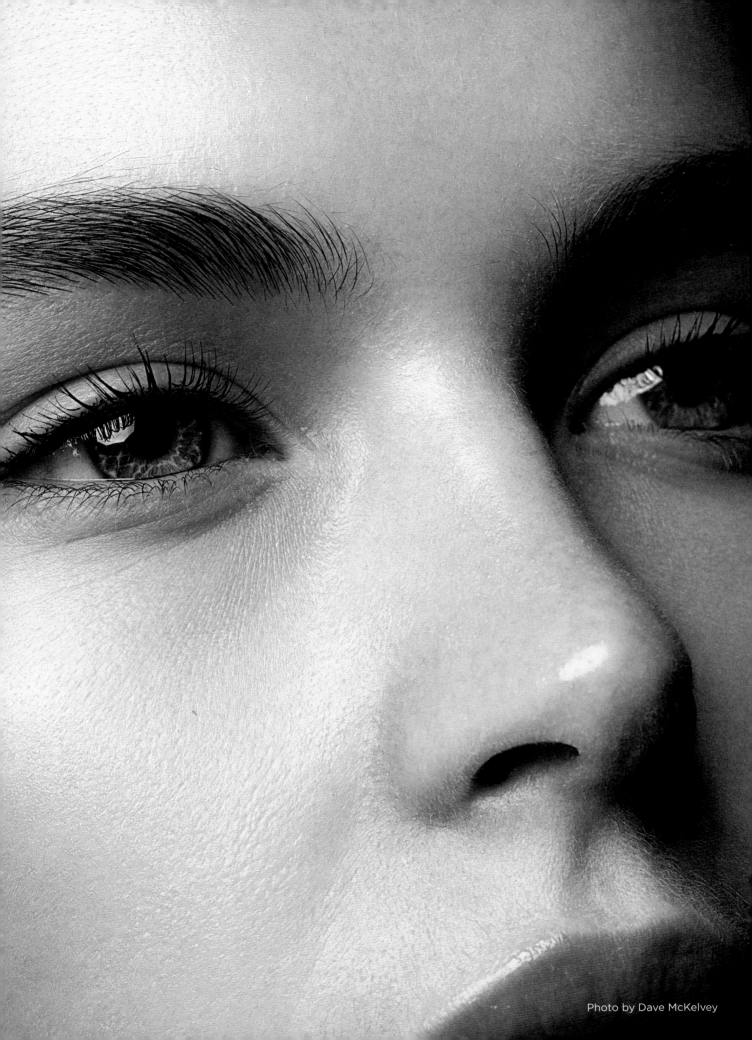

Photo by Dave McKelvey

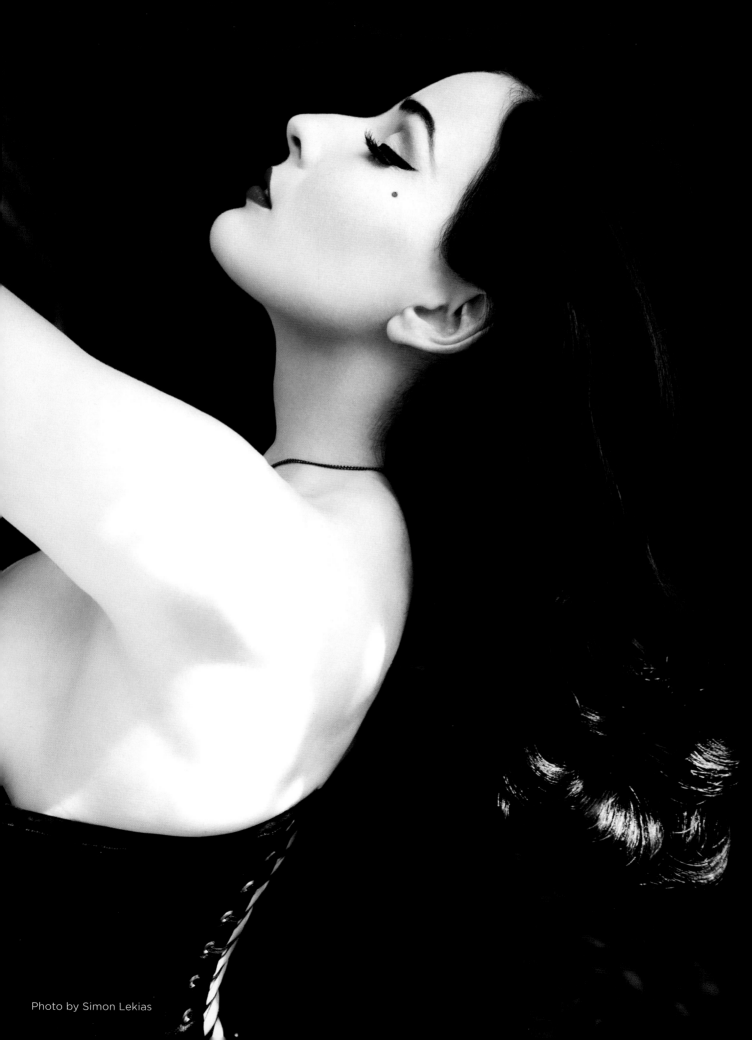

Photo by Simon Lekias

Taming of the brow

Here are the crucial steps to creating beautiful brows:

1. To find the ideal brow length for your face, draw an imaginary line from the outer edge of your nostril straight up to the beginning of your brow. This is where your brows should start. Brows either too close together or too far apart upset the whole balance of the face.

2. Next, while looking straight ahead, draw an imaginary line from the outer edge of the nose, skimming past the outer edge of the iris (the coloured part of your eye) until it meets the brow. This should be the highest point of the brow (the arch).

3. Last, draw a line from the outer edge of the nose past the outer edge of the eye to the brow and this is where the brow should end.

4. Tidy up the brows using slant tweezers, plucking out stray hairs from under the brow. While holding the skin taut, grasp the hair close to the base and pull downwards.

5. Using either an eyebrow brush, a clean mascara wand or a small toothbrush, brush the eyebrow hair downward. You'll see some small, fine hairs. With an eyebrow pencil one or two shades lighter than your natural brow colour, draw a line along the top of the eyebrow as far as the arch with small, feathery strokes. Now, brush the brow back into place, again using feathery strokes to draw a line in the eyebrow from the arch to the ideal end of the brow.

6. Finally, use a brow brush or brow gel to brush the brow hair in an upward direction. Skim your thumb along the top of the brow to turn down any extra-long hairs.

You've now mastered one of the most powerful makeup essentials — a well-groomed brow!

Tip

A baby toothbrush makes a great brow brush. Brush your brows after makeup to remove any powder they may have picked up, then brush upwards and outwards for a polished finish.

Troubleshooting

- To achieve the perfect brow shape, make an appointment with an eyebrow specialist. Most offer a combination of waxing, plucking and dyeing to achieve the perfectly shaped brow. Investigate threading, an Indian method of removing brow hair, where a thread is twisted around the hair, which in turn pulls it out.
- If your brows seem too heavy, try lightening them a couple of shades instead of over-plucking. This softens the overall appearance.
- Remember: a brow pencil is used to enhance the shape of your brows, not to add colour. If you feel your brows need more colour, have them tinted by a beautician. It takes about 10 minutes and lasts about four weeks.
- If you're new to the brow-grooming thing and feel unsure of which hairs should be sent packing, place concealer on the ones to go, stand back, look in the mirror to see if your brows looks better, and then get going. With plucking, less is always more.
- This technique also applies for those considering lightening their brows. Use a clean mascara brush with some concealer applied to it. Brush it onto the brows to get an idea of what the lightened brows will look like.
- If you have already over-plucked your brows, let them grow back — which means zero plucking for around four to six weeks before trying to shape them again. Using a hair growth enhancer is also a good idea.

Tip

Always brush your brows into place after you've applied the rest of your makeup.

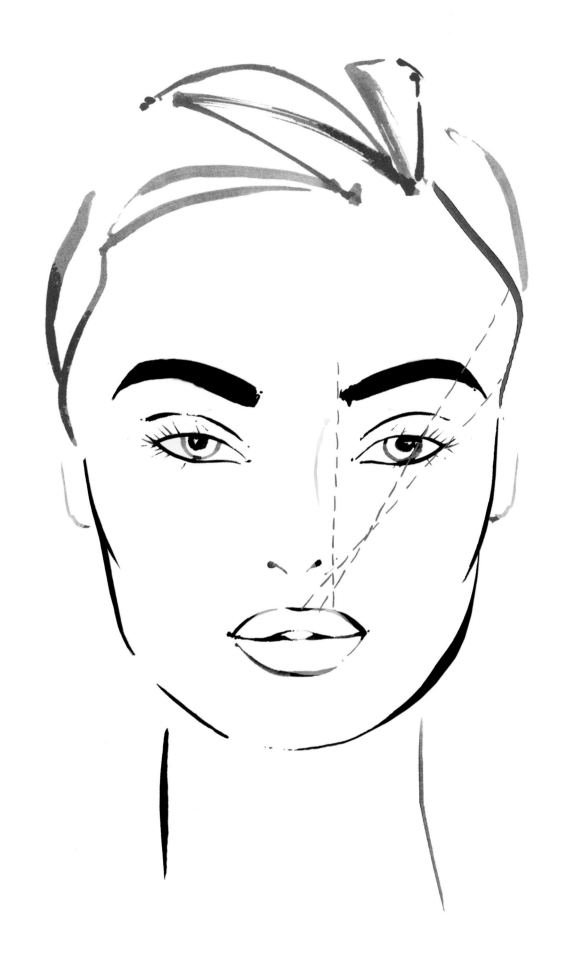

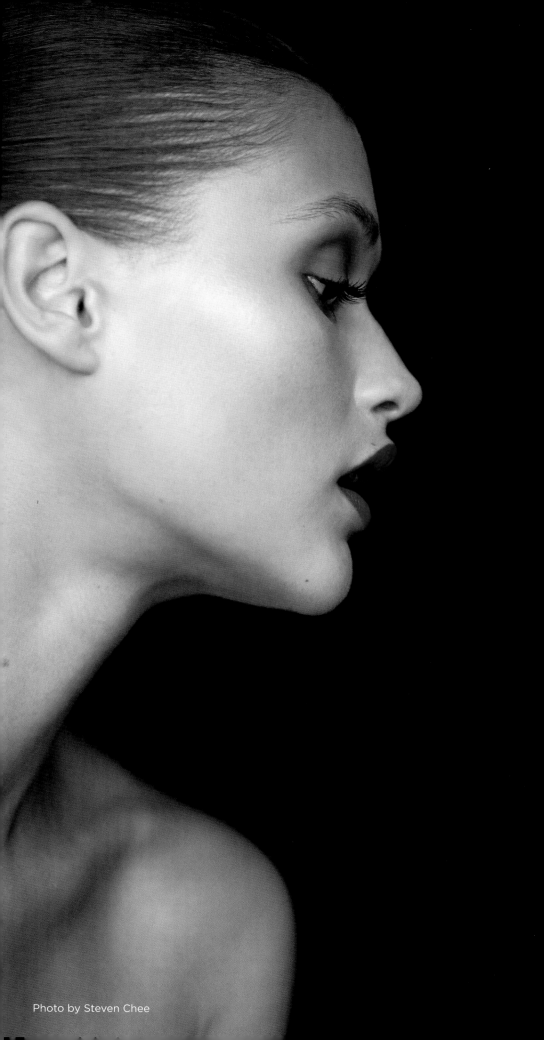

Beauty to me is about being comfortable in your own skin. That, or a kick-ass red lipstick

— *GWYNETH PALTROW*

Eyeliner
— straight down the line

Eyeliner is probably the most versatile of all makeup products. It created signature looks for Brigitte Bardot and Audrey Hepburn, and it's the basis for many eye makeup styles. Eyeliner never goes out of style — it just changes ever so slightly. Don't be afraid to experiment. Anyone can wear eyeliner. Tweak it according to your eye shape. The classic Audrey Hepburn may have a double flick one season and the Brigitte Bardot may take on a metallic twist, but once you have mastered the basics, feel free to try out different looks.

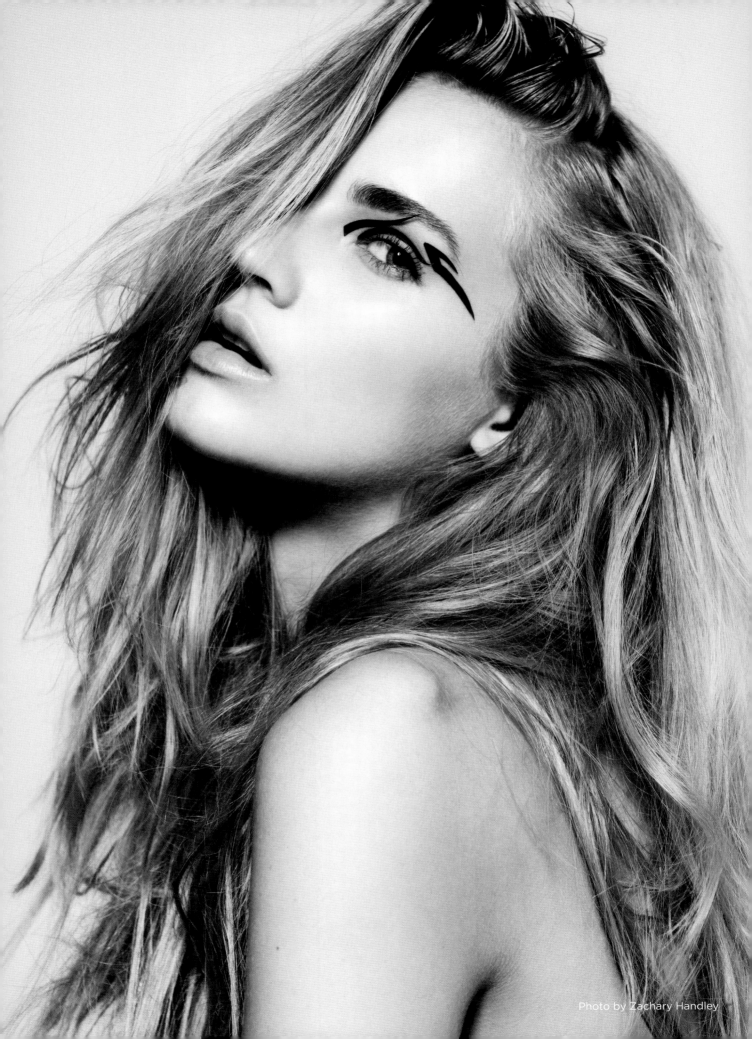

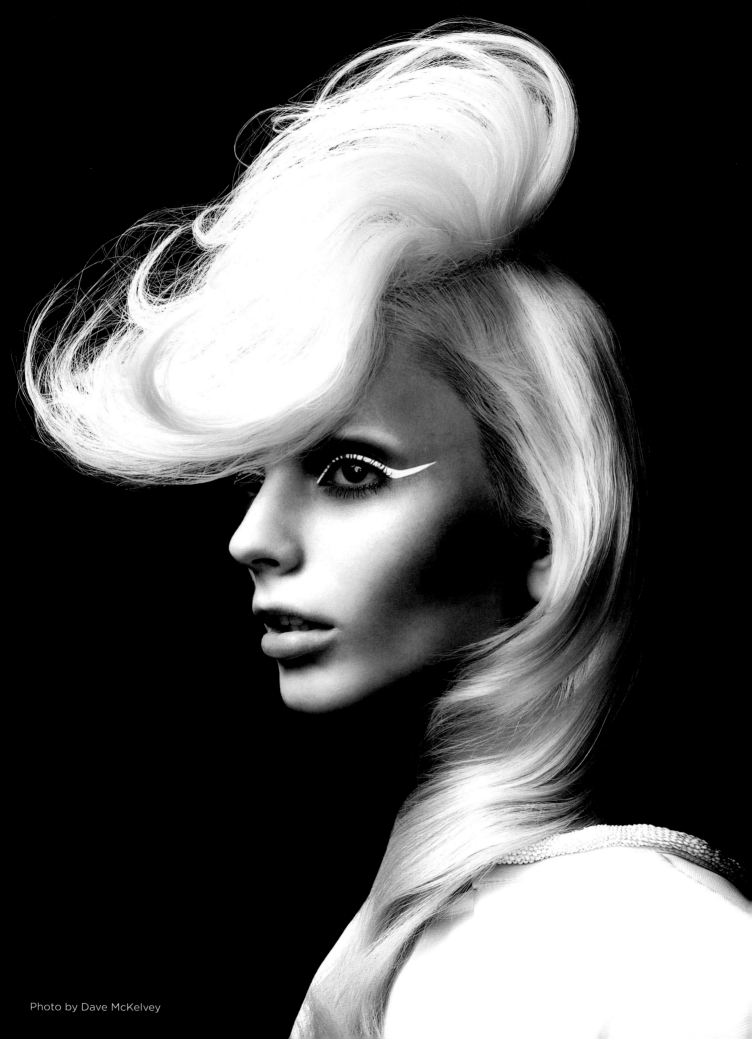

Photo by Dave McKelvey

The line-up

- **PENCILS** These come in varying degrees of stiffness. I prefer soft pencils because they are gentler on the eye and smudge easily.
- **GEL LINER** Gel usually comes in a pot and is applied with a fine brush. It's great for winged looks.
- **CAKE LINER** This is dry and applied with a wet brush to create sweeping lines.
- **LIQUID LINER** Liquid comes in a bottle and is applied with a brush.
- **EYESHADOW** Most eyeshadows can also double as a liner when applied with a wet brush.
- **LONG-WEAR EYELINER** Glides on, then sets to last all day.

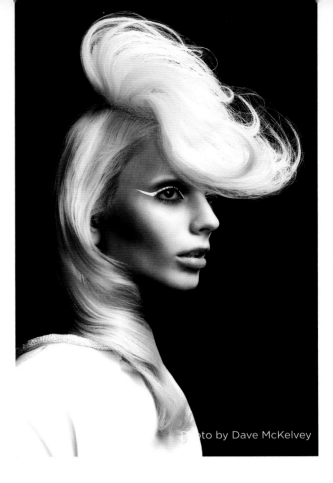

Photo by Dave McKelvey

Troubleshooting

- Always keep your pencils sharpened.
- Shake liquid liner thoroughly before applying.
- If you have a shaky hand, lean your elbow on a table while applying liner or cradle the elbow of your drawing hand with your other hand.
- Don't try to draw one smooth line from start to finish. Use soft, feathery strokes instead.
- Curl lashes after applying liner — they're less likely to get in the way.
- Keep some cotton buds dipped in eye cream on hand to clean up any mishaps or to manipulate the shape of the liner.

Tip

Sharpen eyeliner pencils for more precision and easier application.

The classic liner flick

These looks are pure Hollywood starlet! As with all eyeliner looks, practice really does make perfect.

WHAT YOU NEED

- pencil liner
- sharpener
- small slant brush
- gel or liquid liner
- brown shadow
- lash curler
- mascara
- cotton buds with eye cream or makeup remover (for any mishaps)

STEP BY STEP

1. Starting just shy of the inner upper eyelid, use soft feathery strokes (use a sharpened pencil) to line the eye. Keep the liner even and close to the lashes. Continue three-quarters of the way across the eye.
2. Open your eye and place a dot to mark where you would like your flick to end. If you're unsure, use the tip of your outer lash (with open eyes) as a reference point (see illustration A).
3. Take up where you left off on the lid and draw towards the outer dot.
4. Repeat procedure with the other eye.
5. Looking straight ahead, check eyes in the mirror to make sure the flicks are even.
6. Now you have a rough outline of your flicks, fill in the outer triangle of the line to connect the flick and lashline to give the perfect flick (see illustration B).
7. Blend in the edge of the inner line with a slant brush.
8. For a more intense line, go over the base of the line with liquid or gel liner. This step will also make it more long-wearing.
9. To soften the look, press some matt brown shadow into the line.
10. Curl the lashes and apply mascara.

A.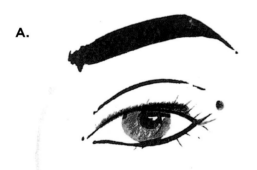

B.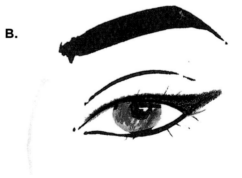

Tip

False lashes work brilliantly here, particularly if you keep the lashes to the outer corner of the eye to complement the flick.

Take it to the next level

Now that you've mastered the classic liner flick, feel free to experiment and customise to make this look your own.

1. Take your look to the next level with this variation by adding liner to the inner rim of the lower and upper lashes.
2. Make sure the bottom liner hooks up with the upper liner at the outer edge and then press shadow into the lashline to add density (see illustration A).
3. Take this look to the max by extending the liner outwards and upwards, and accentuating the feline shape on the inner corner (see illustration B).
4. Curl the lashes and apply mascara to complete the look.

When you master the basics, you can adapt this look to suit any seasonal trend.

Make it personal

Here are some simple rules to finetune, enhance and customise this look to suit your individual eye shape:

- For large round eyes, extend the eyeliner outwards to elongate the eye and make it thicker at the outer corner.
- If you have downturned eyes, start drawing the wing upwards, just shy of the end of your natural lashline. This will give the eyes a lift.
- If you have close-set eyes, start the eyeliner further out to create space between the eyes.
- This isn't the best look for small, hooded eyes but you can adjust it by keeping the line thin and adding lot of individual false lashes.
- If you want an instant eye-lift, keep the rock look to the upper eye and smudge in some dark brown shadow to soften it. The effect of the liner gives back the definition that time has stolen.

A.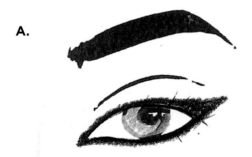

B.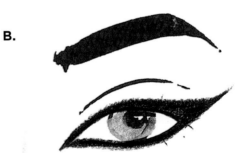

Tip

For the perfect feline flick, first perfect the shape using a slant brush with dark shadow and then cement the flick with liner. Work slowly and gradually build up strength as you go. A little black liner applied to the base of the lashline gives the illusion of thicker lashes.

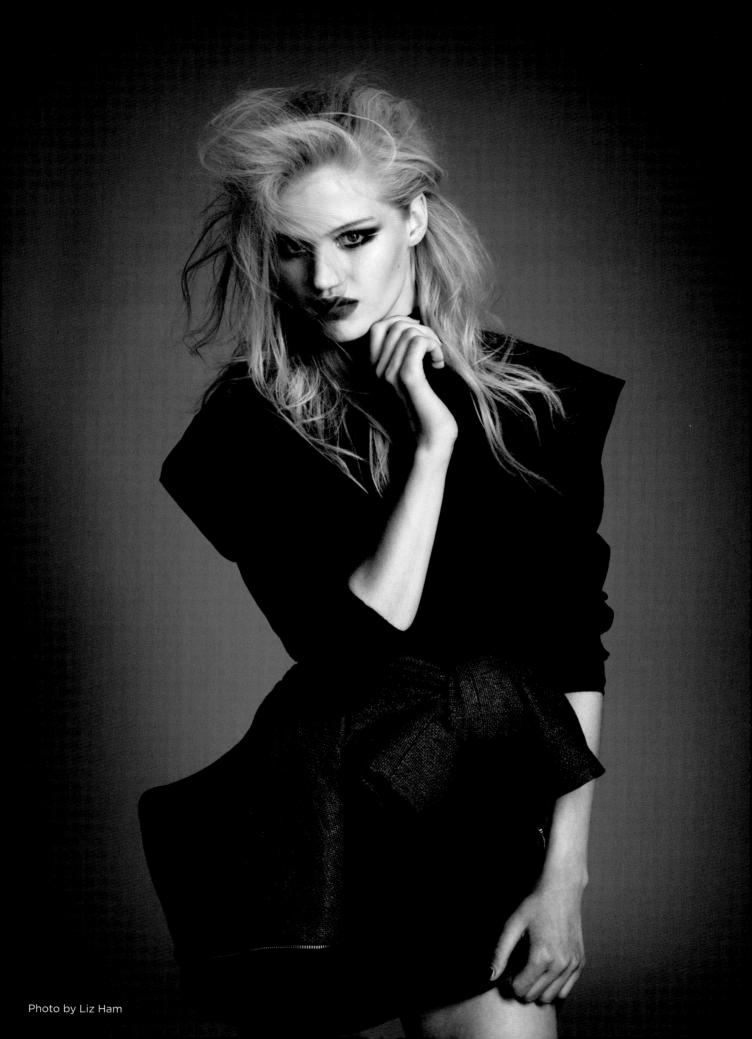

Photo by Liz Ham

I don't think I could live without hair, makeup and styling, let alone be the performer I am. I am a glamour girl through and through. I believe in the glamorous life and I live one

— *LADY GAGA*

The miracle of mascara

The first mascara mixture was concocted by blending coal and petroleum jelly, but it was the invention of the wand that catapulted mascara to the star status it enjoys today. The variations are endless: lengthening, volumising, thickening, curling and defining, to name just a few. So, how to choose? Well, first analyse your lashes and decide what you want your mascara to do. If your lashes are short, go for lengthening mascara; if lashes are sparse, try a thickening one. Remember, you don't have to limit yourself to just one. I often combine two. My favourite combination is one coat of lengthening on the top and bottom lashes, followed by two coats of thickening mascara on upper lashes.

Mascara is available in many different shades, the most popular being black and brown. I like to use black because it gives the most impact and looks the most natural. Some people prefer brown for a 'softer' look, but I'm not a big fan. Coloured versions can be fun and one way to mix things up a little is to use navy.

Mascara is all about impact and when applied properly it really packs a punch, framing the eyes and adding definition. What would we do without it?

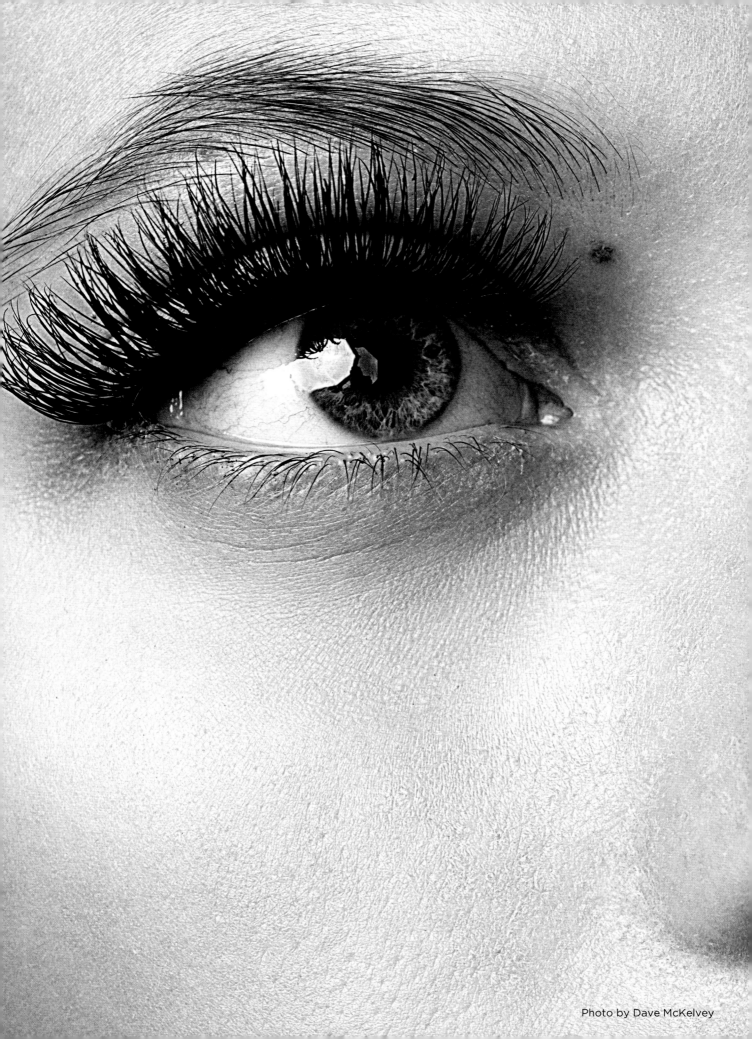

Photo by Dave McKelvey

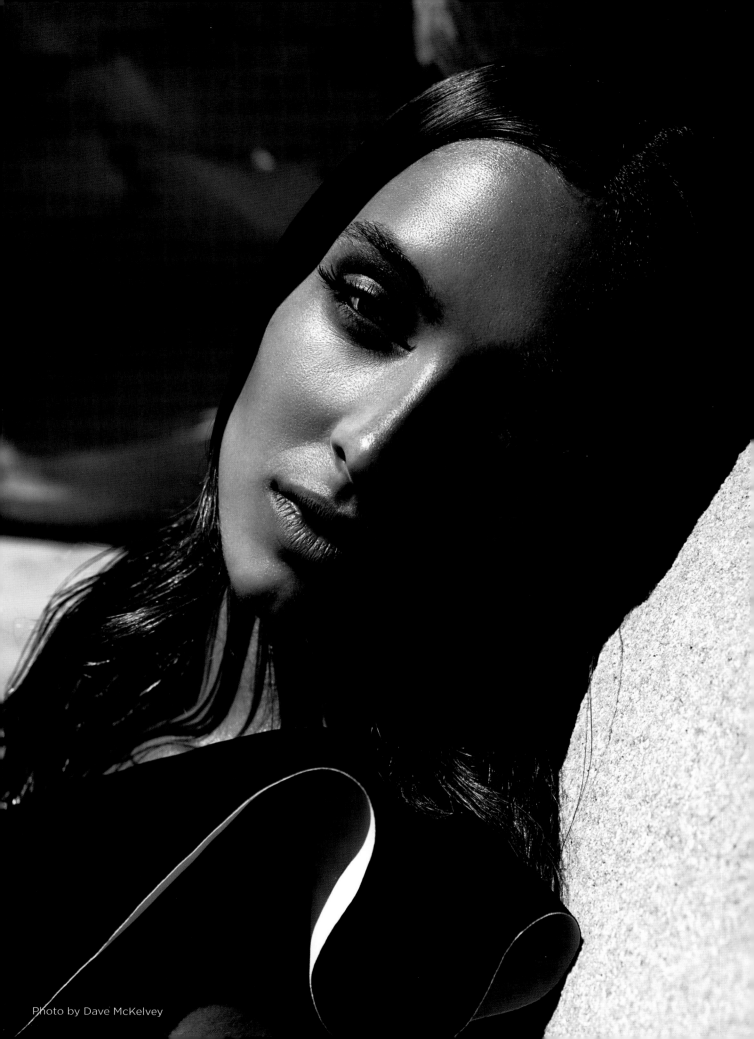

Photo by Dave McKelvey

How to lash out

Here's how to achieve full, sexy lashes every time:

1. Holding the wand vertically, gently brush along the tips of the lower lashes.
2. Holding the wand horizontally, place it at the base of the centre upper lashes and wiggle the brush from side to side.
3. Now that the lashes are sitting in the brush, pull through to the ends.
4. Repeat along the lashline, fanning the centre lashes up and the outer lashes out towards the temple to open up the eye.
5. Have your trusty cotton buds dipped in eye makeup remover at the ready to clean up any mascara mishaps.

Mascara mishaps

SMUDGING

Smudging is the most common pitfall with mascara application. Make sure your lashes are dry before you apply mascara and that no excess eye cream has accidentally strayed onto your lashes. Under-eye concealer needs to be well blended also, because if it's not it can cause mascara to break down and smudge. Another trick is to apply a light dusting of translucent powder where the smudging normally occurs.

FLAKING

Flaking happens when air gets into the mascara tube, often as a result of pumping the wand or not closing the lid properly. However, some flaking occurs because of the lengthening ingredients the mascara contains. Another solution is to apply one coat of lengthening mascara followed by one of thickening mascara.

CLUMPING

If clumping is the issue, allow each coat to dry before applying the next one. Also try lightly blotting the mascara wand before application.

Tips

Avoid smudging mascara by applying it to the bottom lashes first.

Don't pump your mascara wand. It pushes air into the tube and dries it out.

Give your lashes oomph

Falsifying lashes

False lashes first came to fame in the 1930s and '40s with Hollywood actresses such as Marlene Dietrich, Joan Crawford and Bette Davis. Then along came Twiggy in the Swinging Sixties and false lashes became part of everyday life. Falsies are most often associated with high-glamour eye makeup but they do have their subtle side. I use them with almost every look, and the more subtle the look the more important the lash — it's my main tool to emphasise the eyes. When it comes to false lashes today, we are spoilt for choice.

Tip

Curl lashes before applying mascara. It helps open up your eyes.

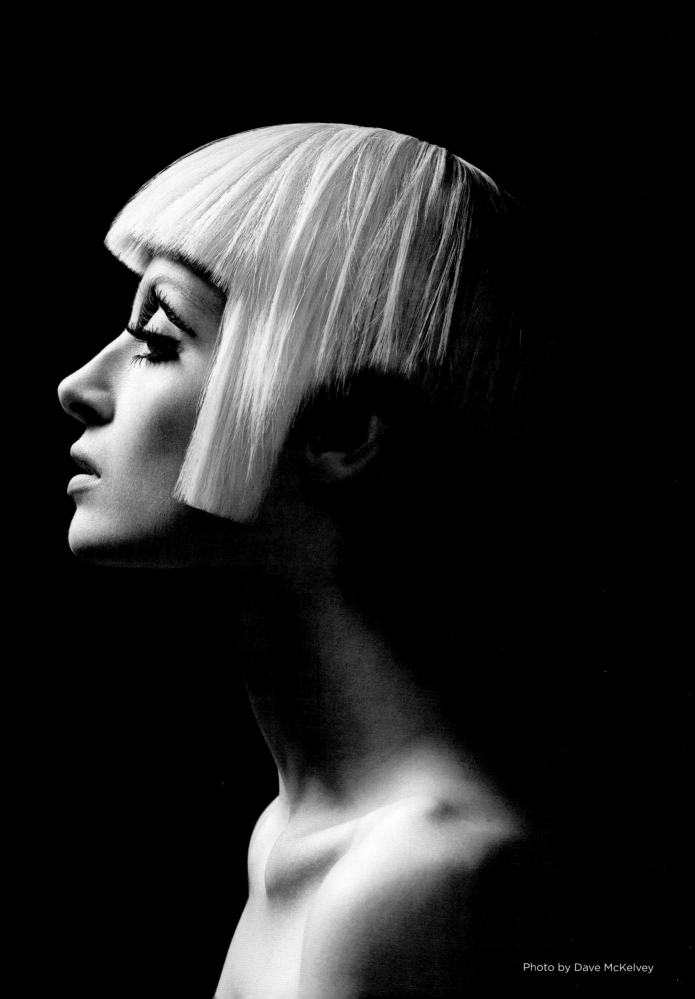

Lashings of style

False lashes come in many varieties. Always use high-quality glue to get the best results. Although some types come with glue, I recommend using duo lash glue. This comes in clear (goes on white then dries clear) or black (goes on black and dries black). I usually work with clear glue, but for very smoky eyes, black works well. You also need slant tweezers and scissors for strip lashes.

INDIVIDUAL LASHES have five hairs sprouting from one fixed point. These are the most versatile and suit everyone.

HOW TO: Apply a small amount of glue to the back of your hand and wait 30 seconds to allow glue to go tacky. Using tweezers, pick a lash from the packet. Ever so lightly dip the base of the lash into the glue. Starting just in from the outer corner of the eye, gently place the lash at the base of your natural lashline. Use the reverse end of the tweezers to lightly tap the lash down so that it sits with your own lashes. Repeat this process until you get to the centre of the eye. Finally, switch to shorter individual lashes for the inner half of the eye.

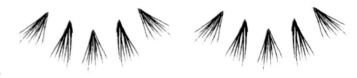

STRIP LASHES OR FULL LASHES are held together at the base by a thin strip that's either black or clear. They create a full look.

HOW TO: Place the lash against your natural lash (without glue) to measure up. Apply a small amount of glue to the back of your hand, pick up the false lash and, with the tweezers, lightly dip dots of glue all along the strip of the lash. Wait 30 seconds for the glue to go tacky. This is essential: if you apply it too soon, the lashes will slide out of place while drying. With the tweezers, place the lash at the outer corner of the eye and work inwards, placing the base of the false lash on your natural lashline. Finally, use the end of the tweezers to lightly press the false lashes into place.

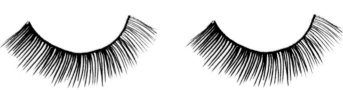

HALF STRIP LASHES give a subtler look and are great with elongated eyeliner or just to accentuate eye makeup.

HOW TO: Apply using the same method as for strip lashes to the outer corner of the eye only.

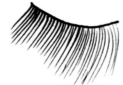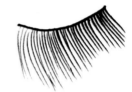

FULL LASH SET IN SEGMENTS (four or five segments) gives the same effect as a full set but is much easier to handle. This method is great for first-time users of strip lashes.

HOW TO: Apply using the same method as for strip lashes one section at a time, starting at the outer corner of the eye.

FRINGE LASHES consist of a long strip of lashes that can be cut to desired length depending on the required look. These are all about the correct trim, so I wouldn't recommend them to a falsie novice.

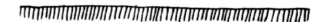

Troubleshooting

- Curl lashes and apply mascara before you start applying false eyelashes. Although you can apply afterwards, it's much easier to get mascara right down at the base of the lashes before you apply falsies.
- Individual lashes come in short, medium and long. Mix the lengths for a more natural look.
- Allow lash glue to feel tacky before placing the lash.
- False lashes, particularly strip lashes, should never extend past your natural lashline — it makes eyes appear droopy.

- If you have droopy eyes, applying a heavier lash towards the outer corner of the eye, stopping just short of your natural lashline, gives eyes a little lift.
- You know you've applied too much glue if it oozes out from under the lash. If this happens, you can wipe off the excess with eye-makeup remover and try again.
- When applying half strip lashes, apply liner to the base of the lashes to make the join invisible.

Tips

For super-easy false lashes, try cutting the strip into three. Use tweezers to put the cut strips in place and make sure you allow the glue to go tacky before applying; this helps the lashes cement straight away to your own.

Use a combination of lengths with individual false lashes for a more natural-looking result.

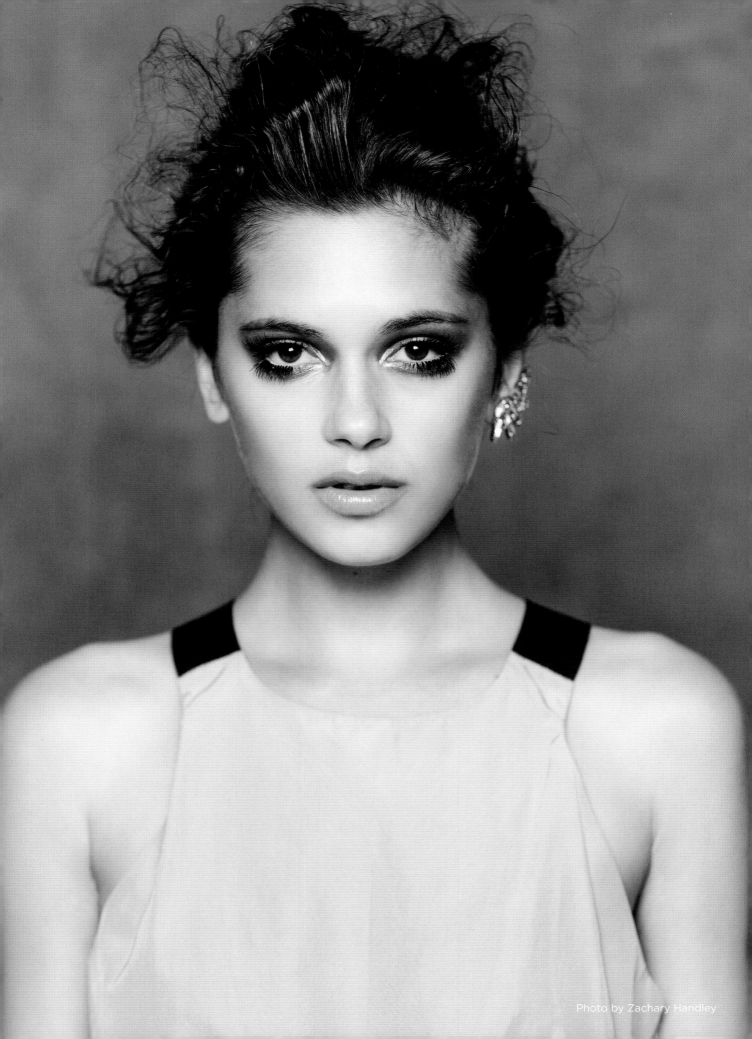

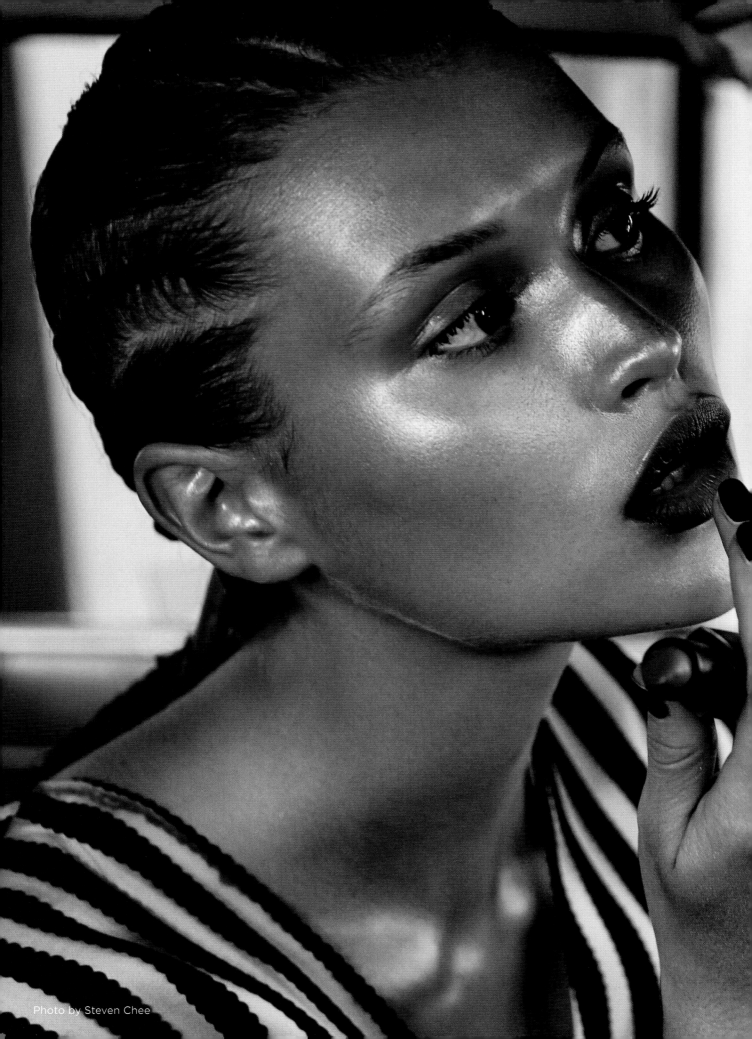

Photo by Steven Chee

I like to drive with my knees. Otherwise, how can I put on my lipstick and talk on the phone?

— *SHARON STONE*

Eyeshadow
— the ever-blending story

Blend, blend, blend. This is the buzz phrase when it comes to eyeshadow. If you're devoid of makeup brushes, do yourself a favour and invest in at least three right now. Choose a long-haired blending brush for blending out shadow; a slightly smaller shadow brush for applying shadow; and a pointer brush for precision application. You'll be amazed at how expertly you can apply eyeshadow with the right brushes.

Another important point is not to overly complicate things. Use a maximum of three or four colours per look — more and you'll have problems blending and your eyelids may seem too 'product heavy'. Keep it simple. Think about the look you want to achieve and how you're going to adapt it to your eye shape.

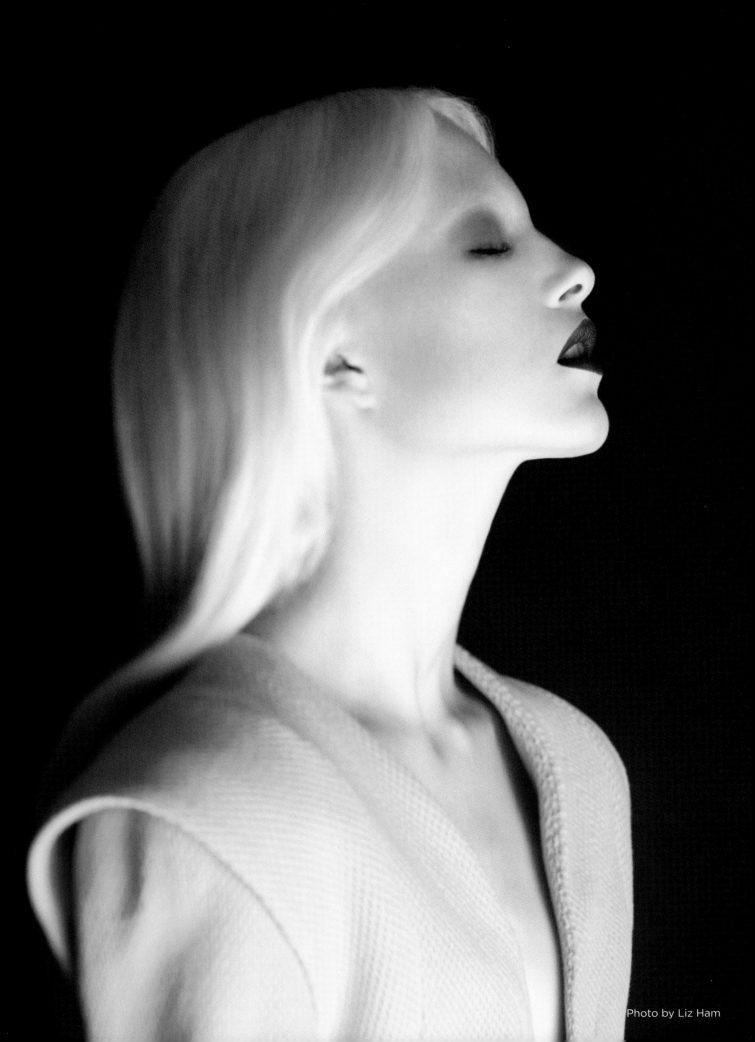

Photo by Liz Ham

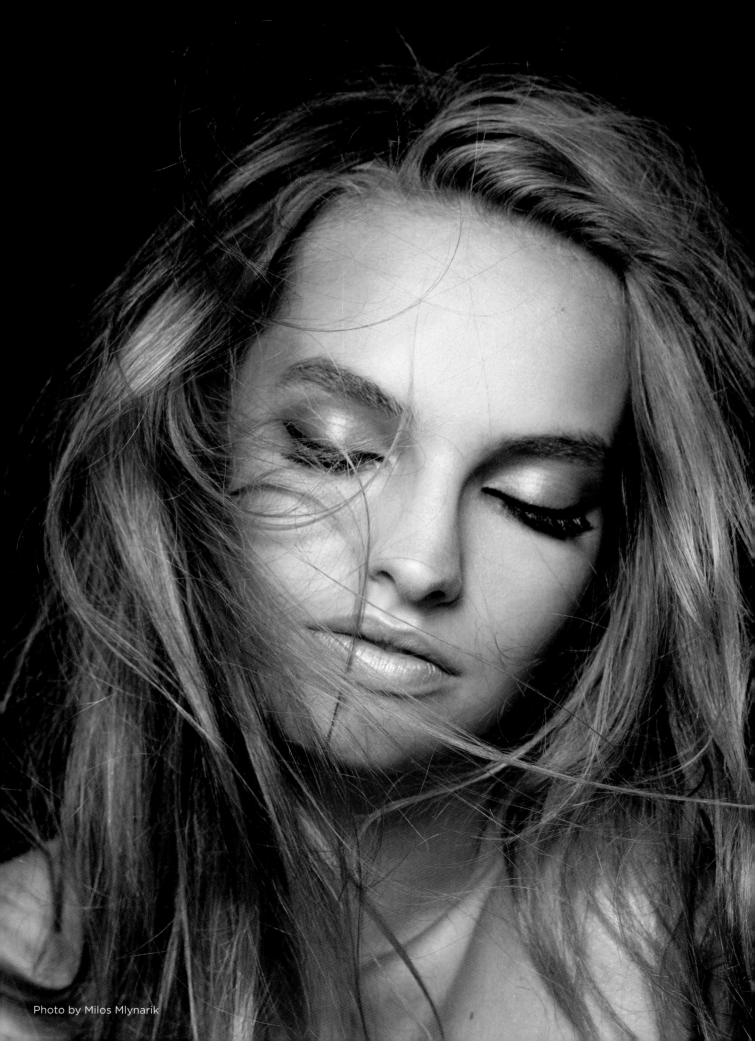

Texture and finish

• **CREAM SHADOW** — goes on creamy, stays on creamy. Apply with fingers to the lid or as a highlight to the inner corner of the eyes.

• **SELF-SETTING CREAM SHADOW** — also known as cream-to-dry shadow or long-wear cream shadow, it goes on creamy then sets to become very long-wearing. I use these shadows as a base coat to the eye. Apply with your fingers and blend the edges with a brush. Work quickly with these to make blending easier.

• **POWDER SHADOW** — this classic eyeshadow comes in endless finishes and colours. It's best applied with a brush. Matt colours are great for definition while satin finishes bring light to the eyes. Try dabbing some metallic shadow onto the centre of the lid with your finger to add a little more drama.

• **SHADOW CRAYONS** — a great invention. They glide on and are self-setting, making them both easy to wear and long-wearing.

Tips

Use a self-setting cream eyeshadow under your powder shadow for super staying power.

Adding a hint of light cream shadow to the inner corner of the eye brings light to the eyes and makes them 'pop'.

On the model opposite I started with a cream shadow, smoked it up with some matt shadow and, to add texture, I dabbed some metallic satin finish shadow to the centre of the lids.

How to shadow to your eye shape

While some tones of eyeshadow will make your eyes 'pop' more than others, it's the placement of the shadow that's really going to define your eyes. Every face is different and changes slightly over time, but here's a rough guide to creating sensational eyes at every age and stage.

CLOSE-SET

Ideally, the width between your eyes should be equal to the width of your eye. If yours is smaller, you've got close-set eyes. Keep darker colours to the outer eyelid and blend outwards. Eyeliner should be applied to the outer eye area and a little highlighter on the inner corners will really open up your eyes.

WIDE-SET

If the space between your eyes is much wider than the width of your eye, you have wide-set eyes. Bring your eyeliner right into the inner corners of the eyes and avoid blending out on the outer corners. Smoky eyes look great on you.

HOODED

Less is more when it comes to hooded eyes. If you want the smoky look, smoke up your lower lashline and place individual lashes on your upper lashline. This will give you an instant lift. Opt for long-wearing liner on upper lashes to avoid your liner travelling.

DEEP-SET

The key to working with deep-set eyes is to bring as much light to the eye as possible, so metallic and satin finishes look great. And don't feel you can't pull off a smoky eye — it's just not true.

DROOPY

The only way is up! Always blend eye makeup upwards and outwards. A great trick is to do your eyes first; then, when you finish, take a cotton bud and a little eye cream and swipe from the outer corner of the eye upwards and outwards to the outer corner of the brow. This gives everything a lovely lift.

ALMOND

If you have almond-shaped eyes, just pick your look and go for it. This is the easiest shape of all.

PROTRUDING

Keep to darker matt colours on the upper lid and lower lashline.

Tips

Use a palette of eyeshadows — you're more likely to get creative.

For beautiful eyes, use long-haired brushes for blending and short-haired brushes for more precision.

The model's eyes were very close-set. To counteract this, first I pulled her eyeshadow outwards and upwards to extend the eyes. I also added a highlight to the inner corner of each eye to accentuate the separation.

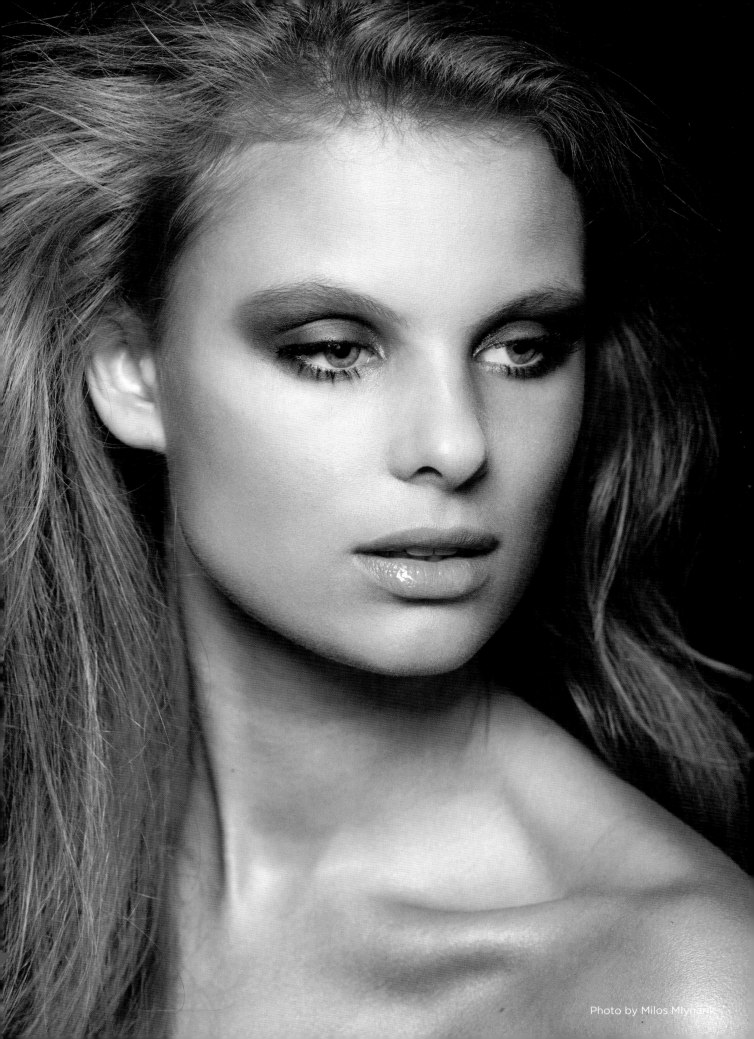

Classic

Looks

Smoky eyes — the never-ending story

The smoky eye is the most sought-after look on the beauty planet. Cream eyeshadow is the easiest way to create a long-lasting look, or you can also use powder shadow for a stronger smoky eye.

There's no rule with the smoky eye — there's so many ways to get there. But the destination should always be that the eye is the main focus.

Tip

Apply smoky eyes before foundation. This way, any mishaps can be easily cleaned up without ruining your base.

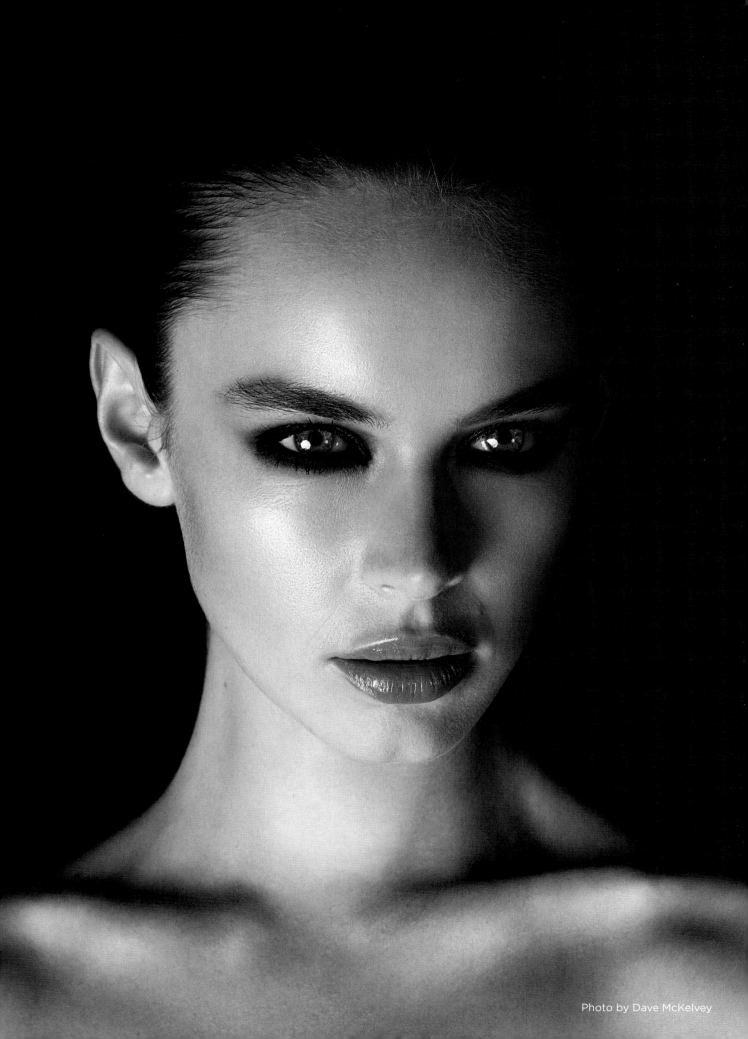

Photo by Dave McKelvey

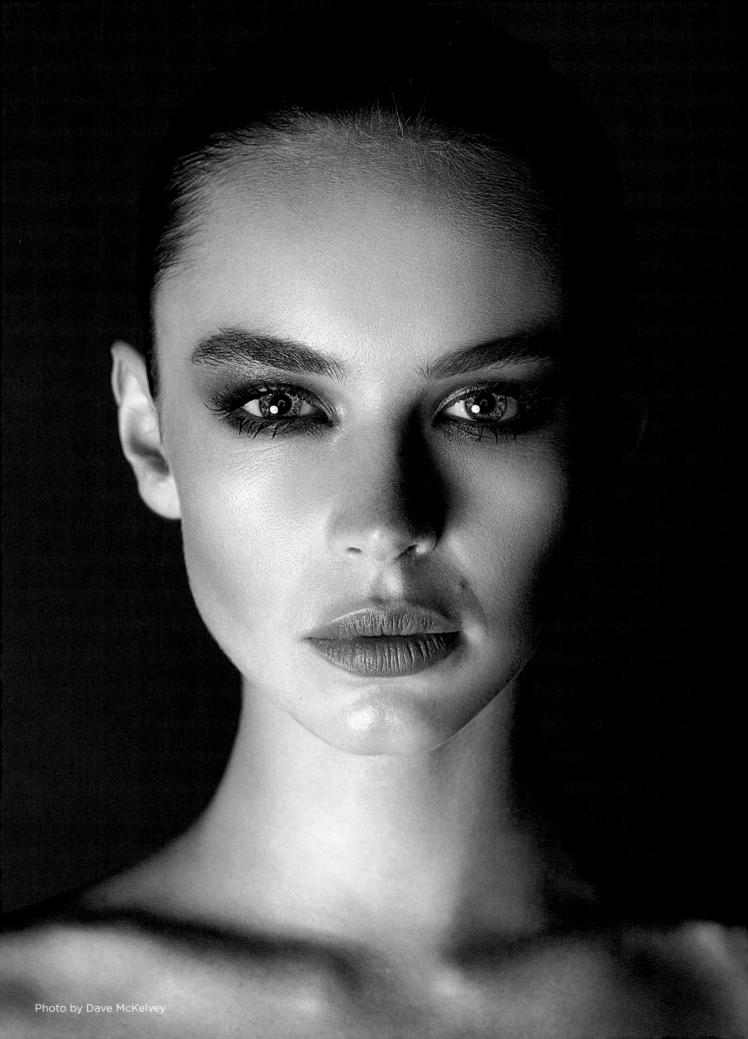

Photo by Dave McKelvey

Smoky eyes with cream shadow

WHAT YOU NEED

- sharpened brown eyeliner pencil
- short-haired pointer brush
- brown cream shadow
- long-haired eye blending brush
- lash curler
- black mascara

STEP BY STEP

1. Using short feathery strokes, apply pencil to the upper and lower lashline, making sure to get right down into the lashes. Then smudge and blend the pencil using the pointer brush (see illustration A).
2. Using your finger, apply the cream shadow to the upper eyelid and blend with the long-haired blending brush.
3. With the short-haired pointer brush, smudge some cream shadow into the lower lashline, paying attention to the outer corner of the eye to ensure the colour on the upper lid and lower lid lines up (see illustration B).
4. Curl lashes and apply mascara.

This is a simple yet really effective technique. For extra oomph, try using a black liner and grey cream shadow. And for those who like a little sparkle, dab a little shimmer shadow on the centre of the lid for a metallic look.

A.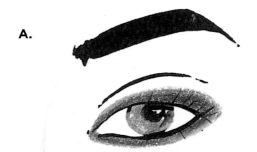

B.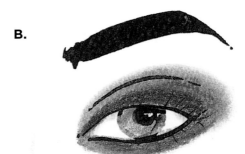

Tip

Work quickly with self-setting cream shadow to avoid it drying before you've finished blending. If it does dry, try a wet cotton bud to buy you a little more time.

Smoky eyes with powder shadow

There are many variations of the smoky eye. This simple version won't take very long to achieve.

WHAT YOU NEED

- soft black liner pencil
- short-haired shadow blending brush
- medium matt grey powder shadow
- short-haired pointer brush
- long-haired eye blending brush
- lash curler
- mascara

STEP BY STEP

1. Apply black liner pencil on the upper lid, starting at the lashline to halfway up the lid using soft feathery strokes (see illustration A).

2. Use your ring finger to soften the stroke and smudge the liner. The natural warmth from your finger makes the blending easier.

3. Use the short-haired blending brush to apply the grey eyeshadow on the lid and up to the crease of the eye.

4. Apply black liner pencil into the lower lashline and smudge with the short-haired pointer brush.

5. Blend some shadow into the lower lashline using the same brush (see illustration B).

6. Using the long-haired eye blending brush, finish off by blending the powder again.

7. Curl lashes and apply mascara.

A.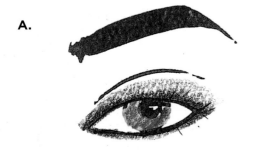

B.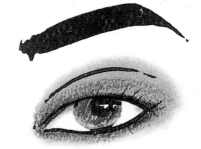

Tip

For a more sultry look, apply liner to the inner upper and lower lashline.

You can apply this technique to any colour. On the model opposite I've used green powder shadow instead of grey.

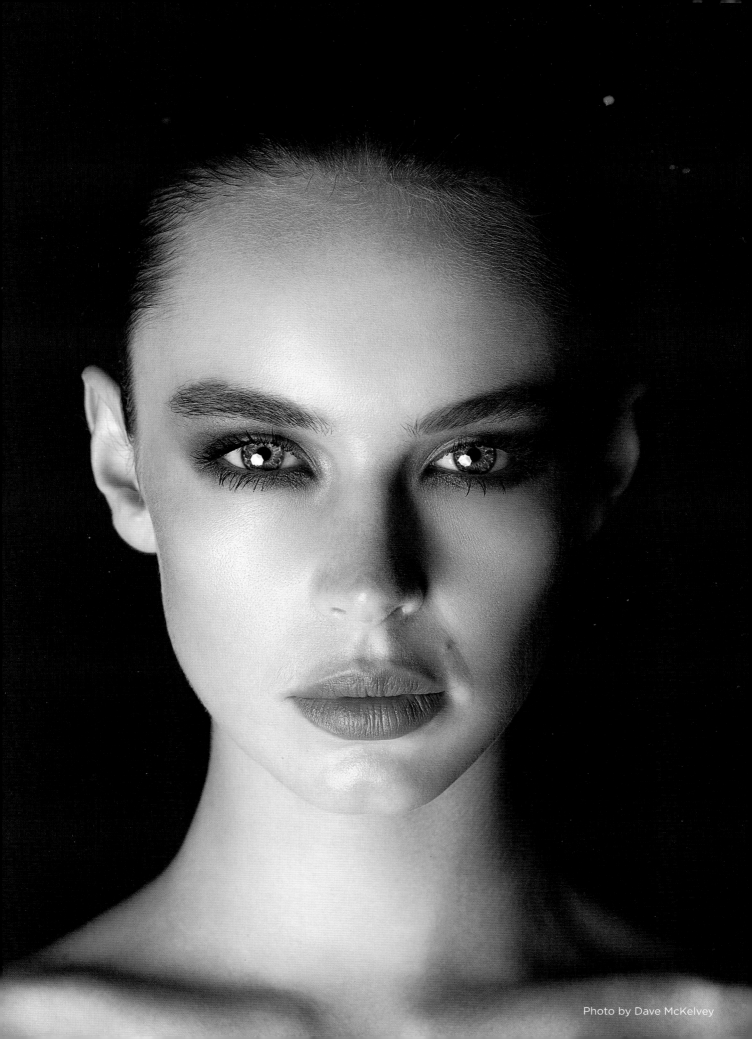

50 shades of red

Absolutely everyone can wear red lips, day or night. They're a great pick-me-up for a tired face and add instant drama to any outfit — and, as an added bonus, they're really easy to apply. You can be red-carpet ready in about five seconds. Many people have an irrational fear of red lipstick, but there is no need. Once you have mastered the correct shade and texture for your skin tone you'll be a convert.

Red lipstick can be broken into warm reds, with an underlying orange tone; cool reds, with an underlying blue tone; and true reds, which are a mixture of both (think the colour of a London post box). If your skin has a red undertone, then you're classified as a cool tone; if it's more yellow, then you have warm-toned skin; and there are a few exceptions to the rule that are neutral-toned. Generally, cool reds look good on cool-toned skin, while orange–reds suit warm-toned skin. True reds suit everyone and neutral skin tones can wear all reds.

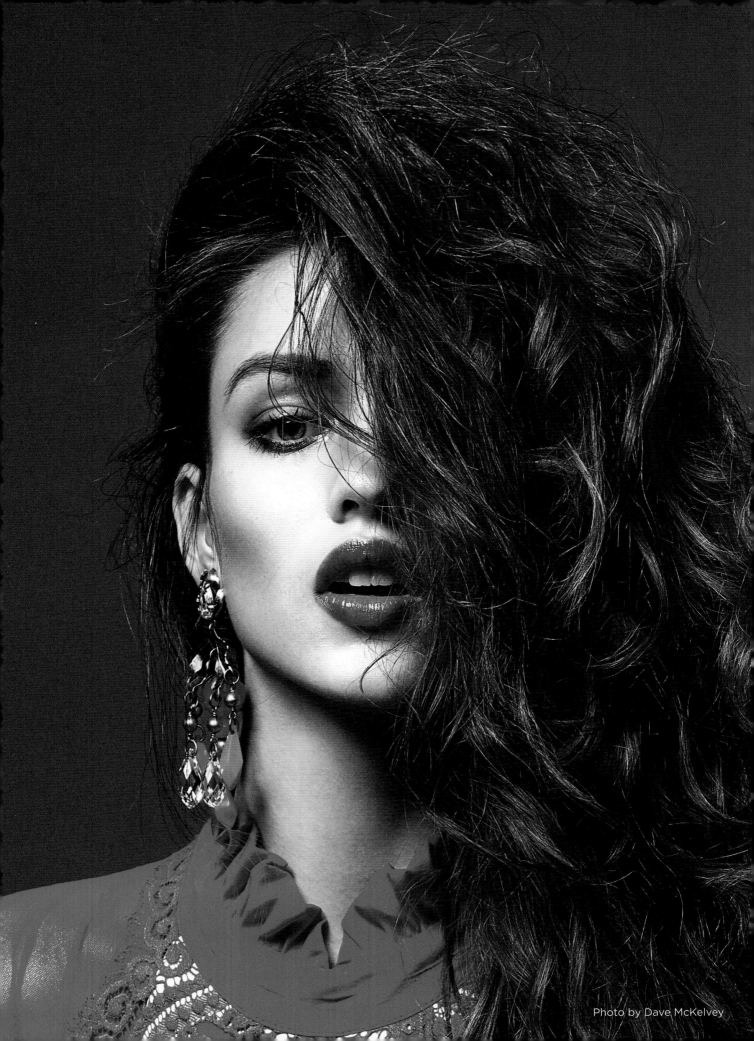

Photo by Dave McKelvey

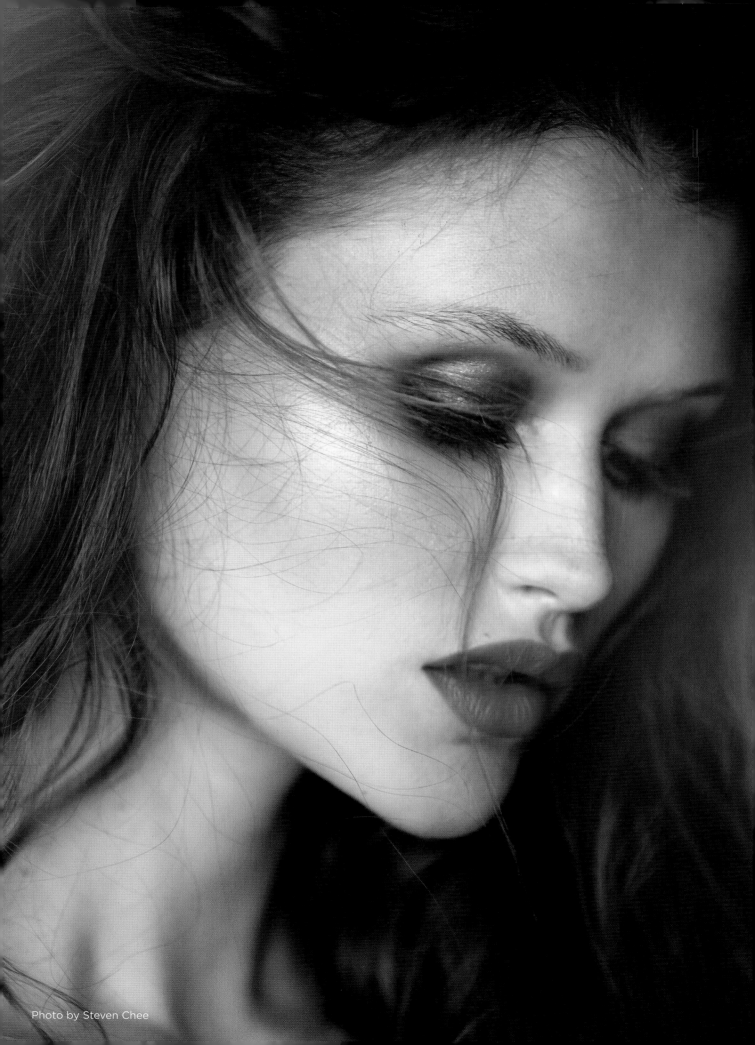

Mix and match

Knowing your ideal red makes the selection process easy. Now you just have to pick the density and finish.

- **STAIN** — a sheer finish, very similar to how your lips would look if you had been eating berries.
- **CREAM** — a creamy dense finish for statement lips.
- **MATT** — a flat finish lipstick to create power lips.
- **SHEER** — a transparent lipstick to create a hint of red.
- **GLOSS** — a coloured gloss that can be worn alone or over lipstick to add a slick of colour.

For intense red lips, apply the lipstick sparingly using a square lip brush. Make sure to press this first coat into every little line of the lips. With a sharpened matching liner pencil, start at the outer corner of the lips and go lightly around the lipline, adjusting the shape where needed. Blot with a tissue and then apply a second coat of lipstick.

Now, wear red with confidence!

Troubleshooting

- Prep your lips by exfoliating and moisturising them before you start your makeup application. Tissue off any excess moisturiser before applying your lipstick.
- You can wear matt red lipstick as a statement or soften it by dabbing it on with your finger.
- To change a creamy-textured lipstick, lightly dust it with translucent powder for a modern matt finish.
- Add a little lip conditioner to your matt lipstick to soften it.
- Blue-based reds have the added bonus of making your teeth appear whiter.

The best thing is to look natural, but it takes makeup to look natural

— *CALVIN KLEIN*

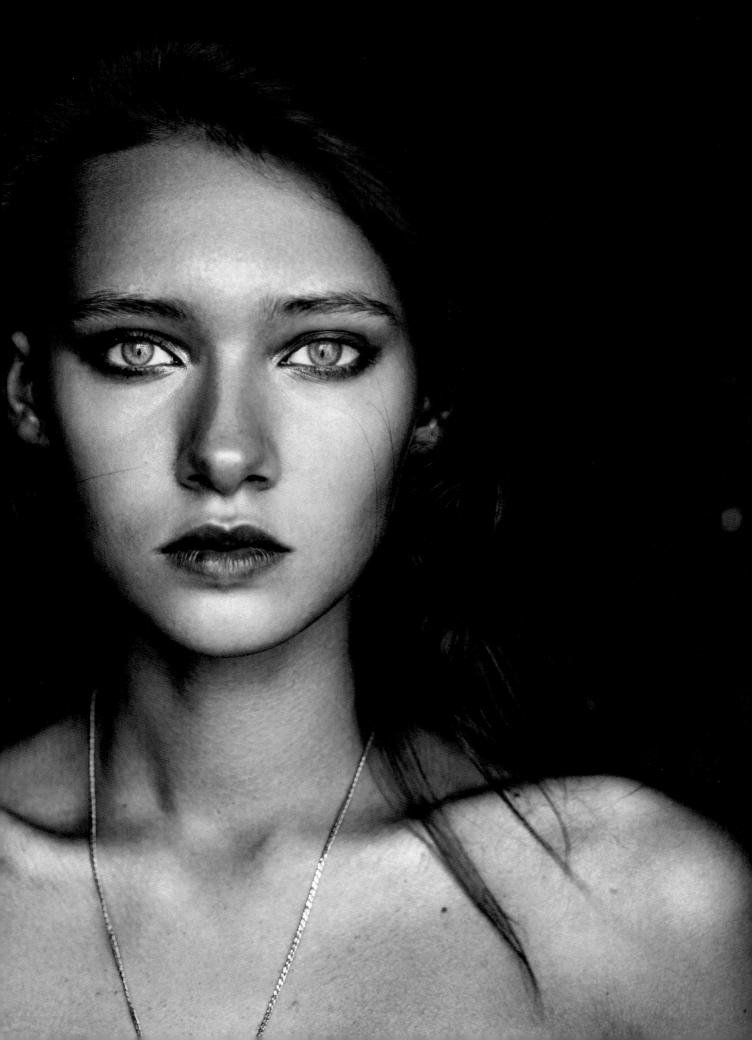

The essential
neutral look

This is a great everyday work makeup created with soft neutral colours that will look refined and sophisticated. You will look made up but without look-at-me smoky eyes or statement red lips.

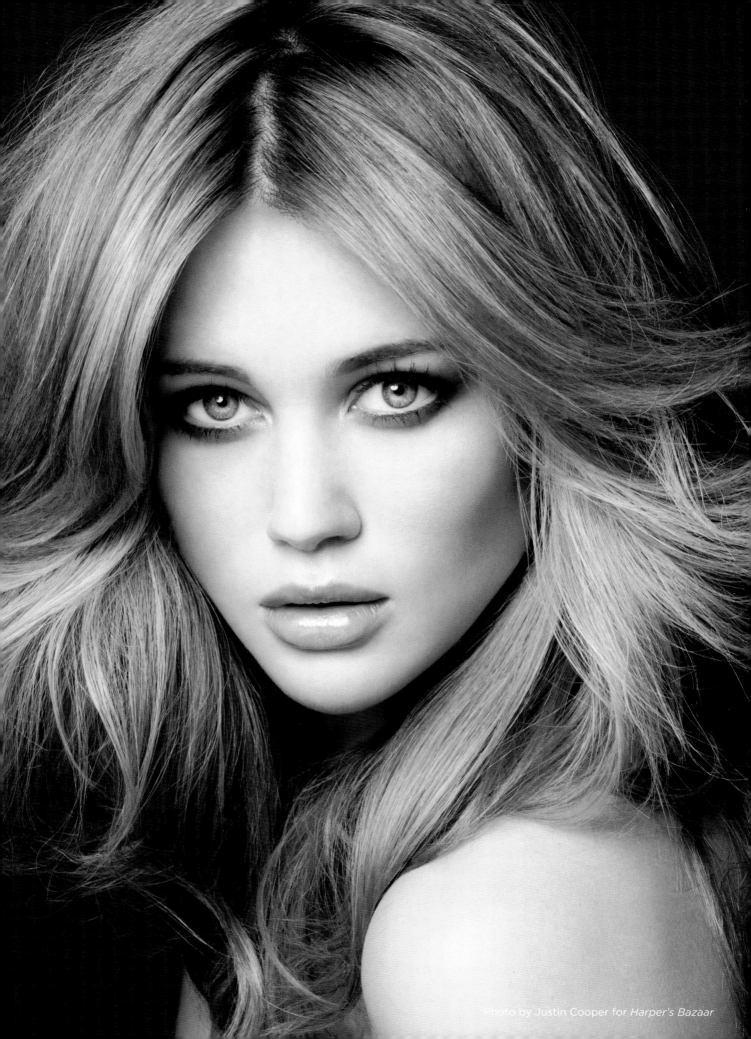

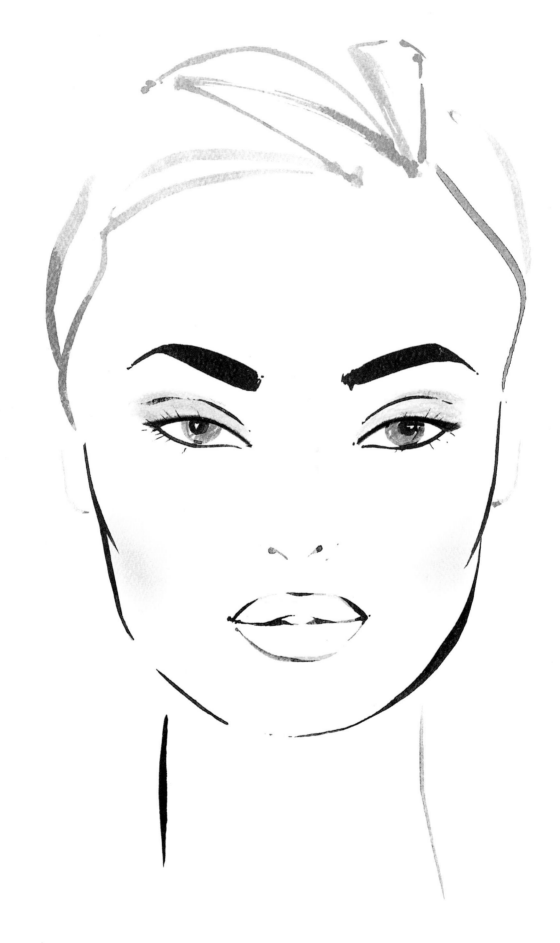

The new neutral

WHAT YOU NEED

- eye cream
- moisturiser
- neutral cream eyeshadow
- long-haired eye blending brush
- foundation
- foundation brush
- translucent powder
- powder puff
- cream contour
- cream blush
- taupe powder eyeshadow
- black liner pencil
- lash curler
- mascara
- highlighter
- brow pencil
- tinted lip conditioner

STEP BY STEP

1. Start with a freshly cleansed face and apply eye cream under the eyes.
2. Apply moisturiser, making sure to spend a few minutes massaging it into the skin. Massaging helps remove any luminosity-zapping dead skin cells as well as improving circulation and skin texture.
3. Using your middle finger, apply cream eyeshadow in mink or slate grey to the lid, from lashline to crease, then blend using a long-haired brush. Allow the area to dry.
4. Starting in the T-zone, blend foundation out to the hairline, then apply translucent powder with a brush to the T-zone or any problem, shiny areas. Finish by pressing the powder into the foundation using a powder puff. This gives a more natural, less-made-up look.
5. Ever so lightly, apply a little contour under the cheekbone and under the chin.
6. Apply cream blush to the apples of the cheeks.
7. Go back to your eyes and, with the long-haired eye blending brush, softly apply some taupe powder to the crease, starting at the outer eye and working in.
8. With a well-sharpened soft black pencil, draw a line into the upper lashline from the outer corner to halfway in. Keep this line as close as you can to the lashline. If the line looks too obvious, smudge it with a brush or cotton tip.
9. Curl lashes and apply two or three coats of mascara to upper lashes and one coat to lower lashes.
10. Add highlighter to cheekbones, the bridge of the nose and lips.
11. Brush and pencil in brows.
12. Last but not least, add a tinted lip conditioner.

Troubleshooting

- Another option is to dab a little bronze or silver shadow only to the centre of the lid.
- Always apply your makeup in good, even lighting.
- Add a few individual false lashes for a special event.

The no-makeup makeup look

The no-makeup look enhances natural features and conceals any flaws, all the while appearing virtually undetectable to the eye. This is a very popular option for runway models because it creates the appearance of a fresh and modern nude face.

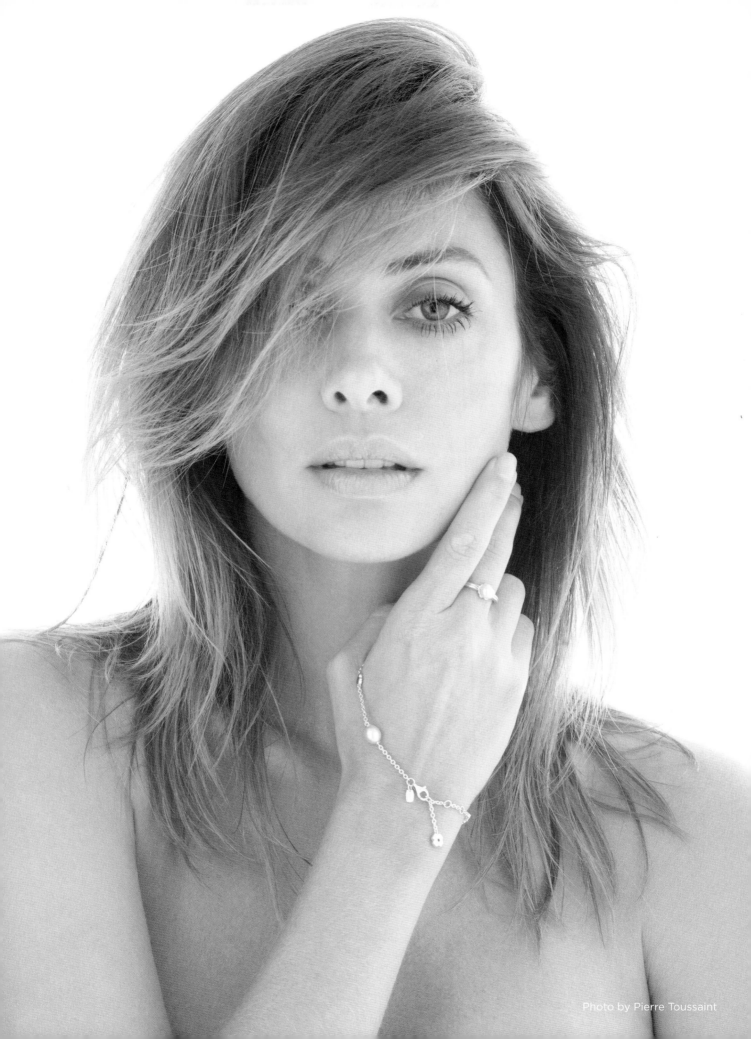

Photo by Pierre Toussaint

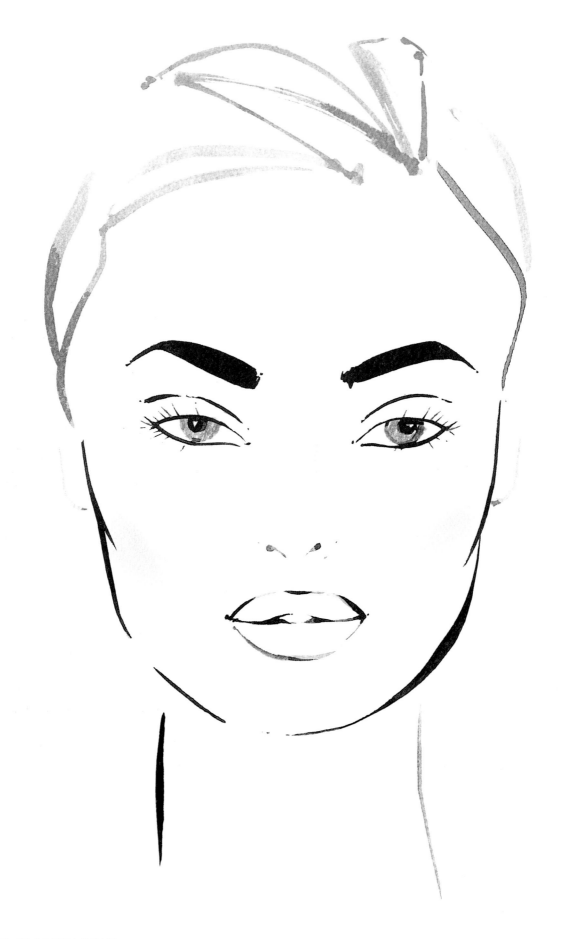

Bare it all

This is a great look to master for those days you don't want to appear to be wearing makeup — think holidays, going to the beach, school — or if you're wearing a very flamboyant outfit and want to balance it out with a modern bare face.

WHAT YOU NEED

- eye cream
- moisturiser
- concealer brush
- concealer
- brow pencil or brow gel
- lash curler
- mascara
- contour
- cheek stain
- foundation brush
- bronzer
- highlighter
- tinted lip conditioner

STEP BY STEP

1. Start with a freshly cleansed face and apply eye cream under the eyes.
2. Apply moisturiser, making sure to spend a few minutes massaging it into the skin. Massaging helps remove any luminosity-zapping dead skin cells as well as improving circulation and skin texture.
3. The nude look is all about precision. Have a good look in the mirror, lower your chin (this will make dark areas look more prominent) and decide what you would like to conceal. Using a concealer brush, apply concealer sparingly to the darkened areas and blend by dabbing lightly with your ring finger.
4. Using your middle finger, apply concealer to any areas that need a little extra help, such as around the nose and inner corner of the upper eye.
5. Pencil in brows to balance out the face or apply a little brow gel to tame unruly brow hair.
6. Apply one coat of your favourite mascara.
7. Apply contour where needed (see page 47).
8. Using a cheek stain and a foundation brush, apply blush to the apples of the cheeks and blend up and back towards the hairline.
9. Use a light dusting of bronzer to the perimeter of the face and a delicately applied highlighter to the cheekbones.
10. Lastly, apply a little tinted lip conditioner and you're on your way.

Troubleshooting

- If you have oily skin or large pores, wear a pore-minimising primer after your moisturiser.
- Make sure your cheek tint and lip conditioner are tonal, or add a little of the cheek tint to the lips followed by a touch of pawpaw cream.

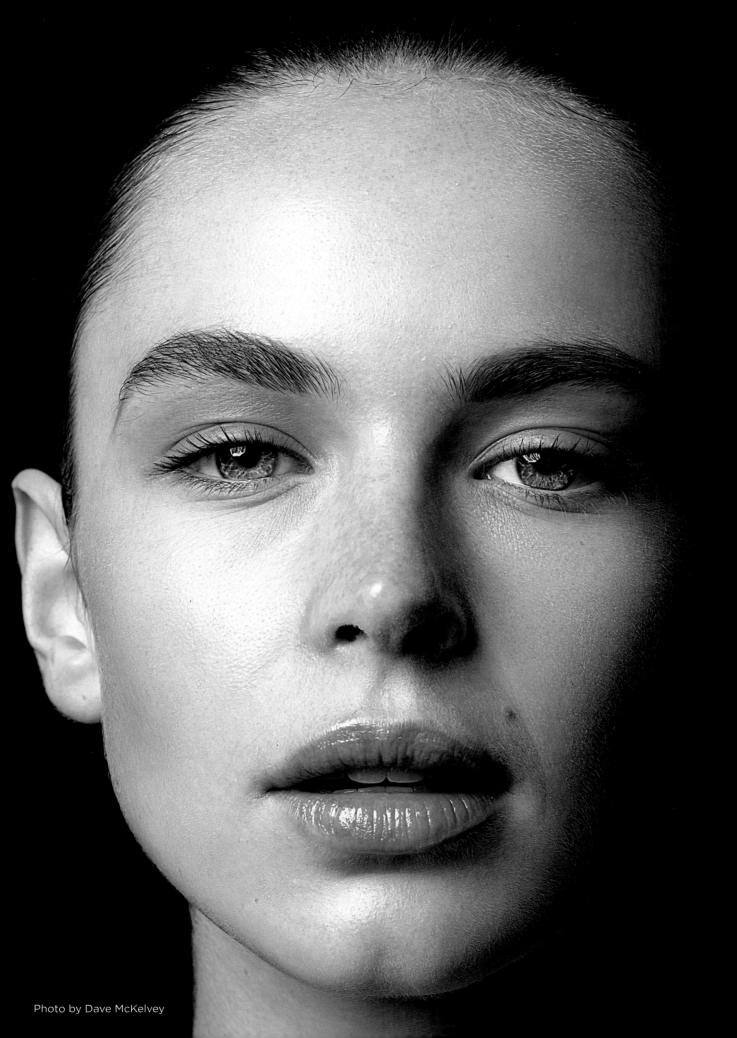

Photo by Dave McKelvey

Nature gives you the face you have at 20; it is up to you to merit the face you have at 50

— COCO CHANEL

Get

the Look

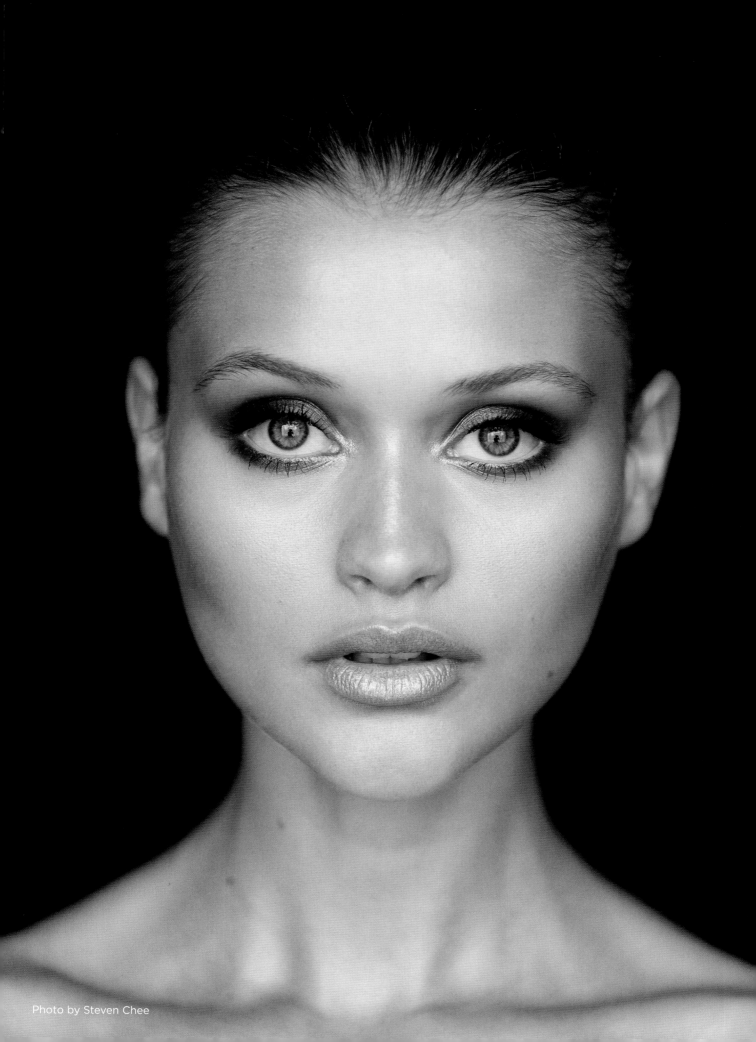

Photo by Steven Chee

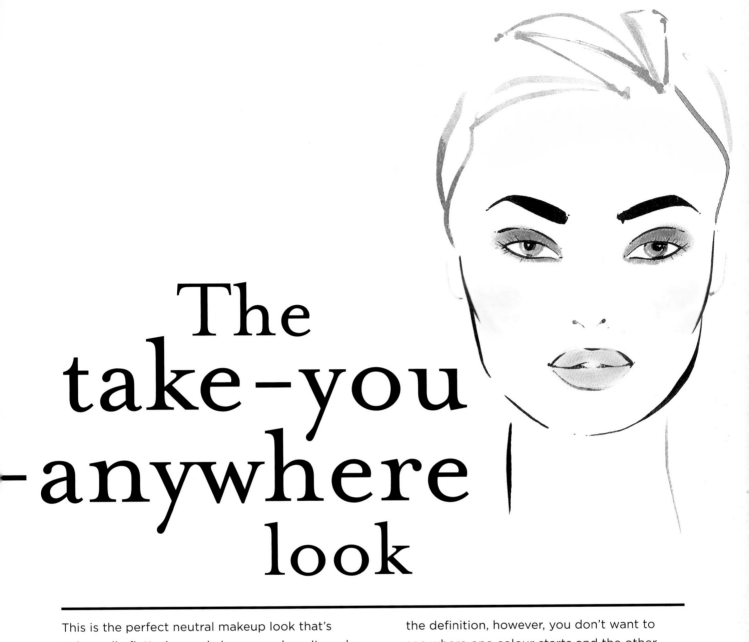

The take-you -anywhere look

This is the perfect neutral makeup look that's universally flattering and always modern. It works just as well on the red carpet as it does in the office.

STEP BY STEP

1. Apply light-brown self-setting cream eyeshadow to the lid and blend into the crease using a long-haired blending brush.
2. With a shadow brush, apply dark gold shadow to the lid and into the crease.
3. Using a pointer brush, smudge some bronze shadow into the lower lashline.
4. Add a little dark brown eyeshadow onto the outer corner of the eye and into the crease.
5. Lightly blend all the colours together using a long-haired blending brush. You still want the definition, however, you don't want to see where one colour starts and the other one ends.
6. Curl the lashes and apply two coats of mascara.
7. Add some individual lashes.
8. Apply brow pencil where needed and brush brows into place.
9. Add some coral-based cream blush to the apples of the cheeks and blend back and up.
10. Lightly contour the hollows of the cheeks.
11. Draw the light to the eyes by adding a soft gold cream eyeshadow to the inner corner of the eyes.
12. Add a hint of luminizer to the cheekbones and Cupid's bow.
13. Finish with a satiny nude lipstick.

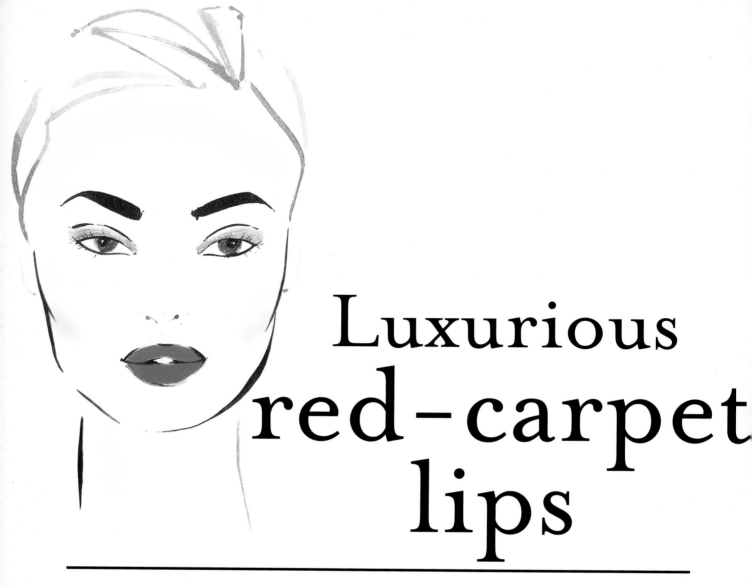

Luxurious red-carpet lips

Red lips are spectacular — but only when done well. For this look, the focus is on a classic blue–red lipstick, which gives great definition to the lips and also makes teeth look whiter. When talking about red lips, it's the age-old beauty question: do I play up eyes or lips? Well, it's all about balance. You will need some definition on the eyes for a red-carpet event. However, you don't want the face to appear too heavily made up.

STEP BY STEP

1. Start with your signature foundation. (To find your perfect match, turn to the chapter on foundation.)
2. Conceal where needed around the base of the nose and the chin, and add powder to the T-zone with a brush.
3. Apply light-brown self-setting cream eyeshadow over the entire lid and blend into the crease.
4. Smudge some brown kohl liner into the upper lashline and set with bronze shadow.
5. Using a shadow brush, apply some light bronze shadow to the lid and then use the same light bronze colour and a pointer brush to apply to the lower lashline.
6. Apply red lipliner to your natural lipline, starting at the outer corners and working inwards, then blend with a lip brush.
7. Fill in the lips using a lip brush coated with the blue–red lipstick.
8. Contour the hollows of the cheeks.
9. Apply cream bronzer to the perimeter of the face with a large bronzer brush.
10. Add a little highlighter to the cheekbones.

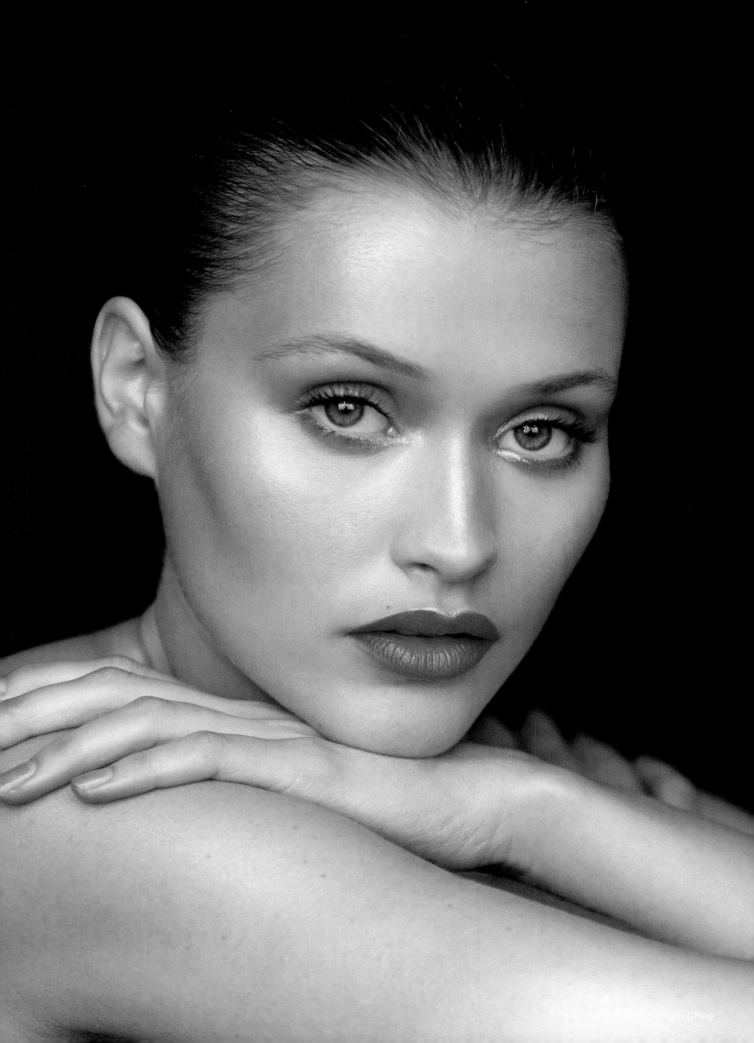

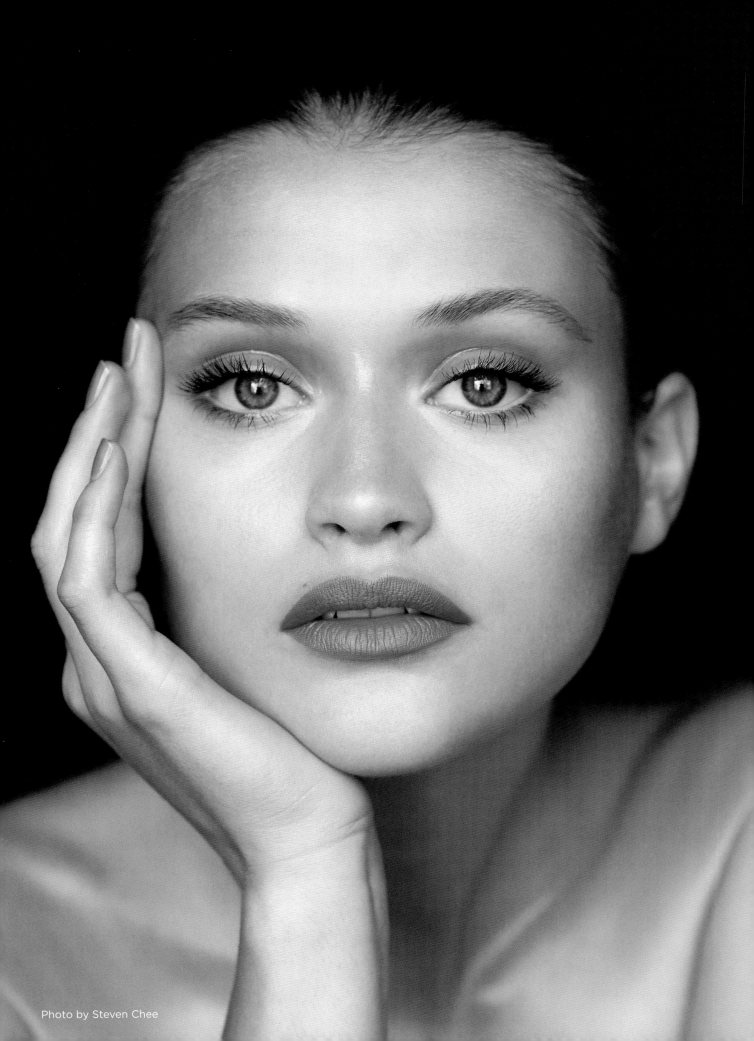

Photo by Steven Chee

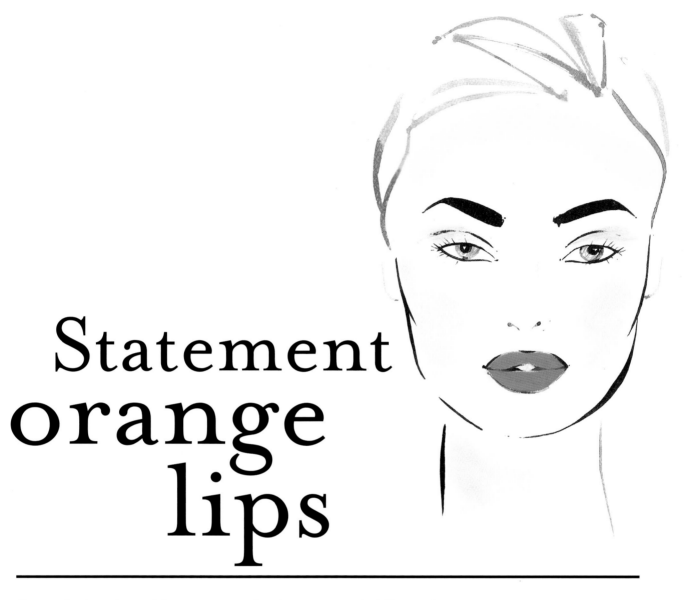

Statement orange lips

Orange is *the* colour of the moment and a nice change from red. These lips say, 'I'm here, I'm polished and I know my style.' The trick to pulling off this colour is to perfect the rest of the look without overwhelming the lips.

STEP BY STEP

1. Apply your signature foundation and concealer where needed.
2. Apply a self-setting cream shadow in a mink shade on the lids and into the crease of the eye.
3. Using a brow pencil one shade lighter than your natural colour, pencil in your brow to add some extra fullness. Remember to draw light, hairlike strokes.
4. Curl lashes with an eyelash curler and apply two coats of mascara.
5. Apply orange lipliner to the natural line of the lips, starting at the outer corner and working your way into the centre.
6. Blend the edges of the lipliner using a lip brush.
7. Apply lipstick using a lip brush, starting at the centre of the lips and working out towards the liner.
8. Add some cream bronzer to the perimeter of the face.

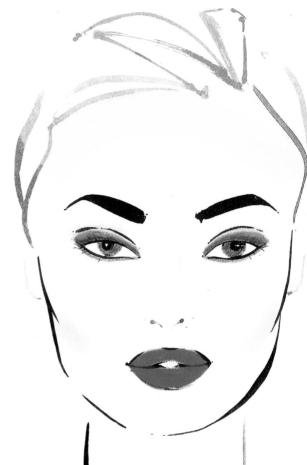

Taking your makeup from day to night

To take you effortlessly from office to bar, you need to plan ahead. Choose a day look that you know you can transform easily by adding to it, rather than having to start all over again.

STEP BY STEP

1. Take off your day lipstick with makeup remover so you have a fresh canvas.
2. Add red lipliner to your natural lipline then blend with a lip brush.
3. Using the same lip brush, apply lipstick, starting in the centre and blending out towards the lipline.
4. Frame the face by brushing on cream bronzer to the perimeter of your face to balance the skin tone against the boldness of the red lips.
5. For a touch more glamour, add luminizer to your cheekbones.

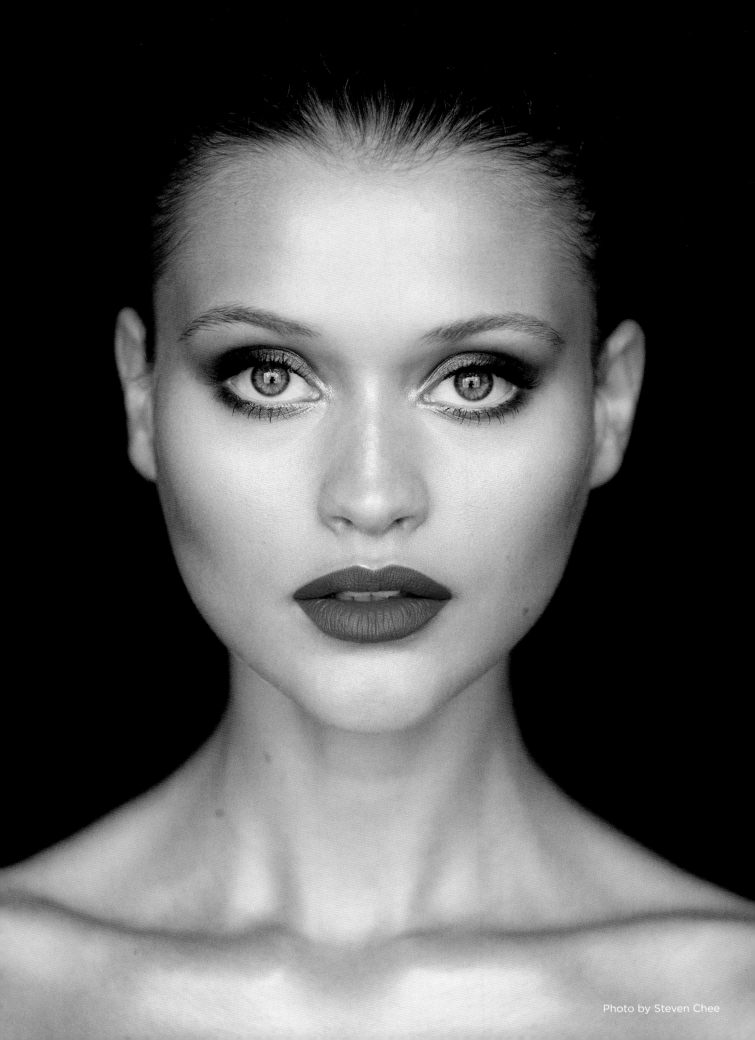

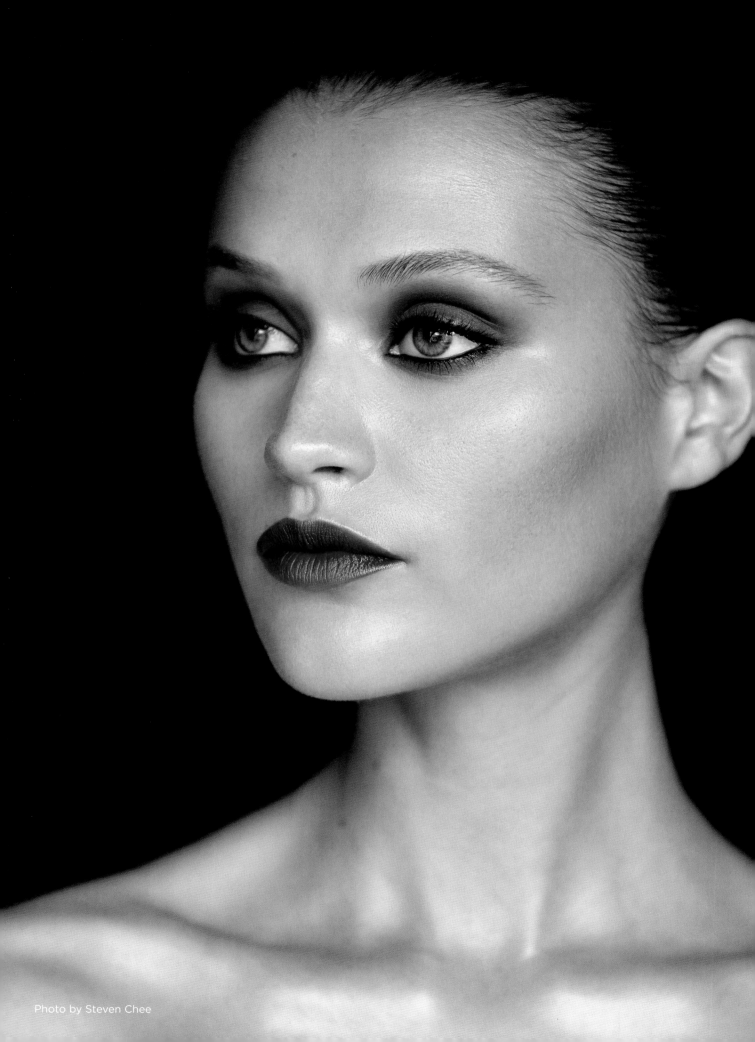

Photo by Steven Chee

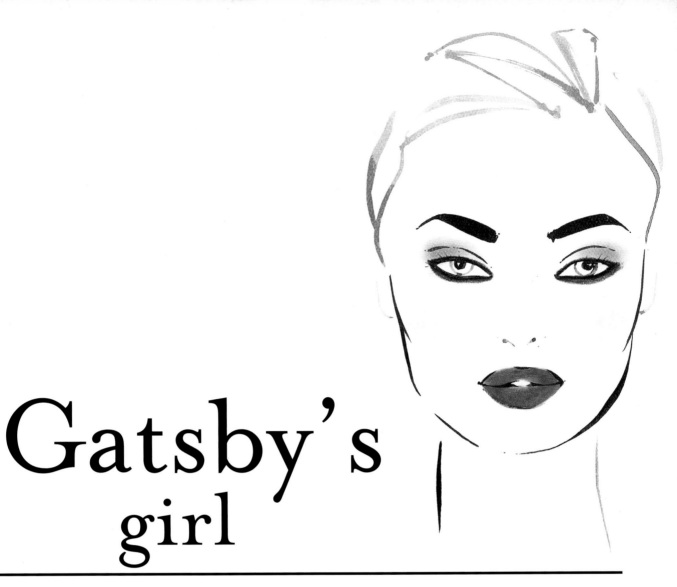

Gatsby's girl

Inspired by the movie, you can take some bold elements of this look or embrace it all. The deep cranberry and berry tones give it a vintage feel.

STEP BY STEP

1. Apply black kohl to the upper and lower waterline (inner lids) of the eyes.
2. Next, add a warm-toned brown cream shadow to the upper lid.
3. Add a dark, wine-coloured shadow to the upper lashline for more depth, applying slightly more depth to the outer corner of the eye.
4. As a finishing touch, add a cranberry-coloured satin-finish shadow into the crease of the eye and into the lower lashline.
5. Curl lashes and apply three coats of mascara.
6. Draw a berry lipliner onto the natural lipline, starting at the outer corner and working your way in.
7. Fill in with a dark berry lipstick and then tissue off so it appears more stain-like.
8. Finish by adding cream bronzer to the perimeter of the face to balance the skin tone against the dark lip.

Tip

Try a sheer berry lip gloss for a softer approach.

The essential eye flick

This is a versatile, eye-defining asset to have in your makeup arsenal. It's easy to tweak to suit individual eye shapes.

STEP BY STEP

1. Using a sharpened black eyeliner pencil, line the upper lashline three-quarters of the way along, starting from the inner corner.
2. Mark the point where you would like the flick to end, and draw to that point. If you're unsure, take your cue from the lower lashline. Draw an imaginary line to the end of your brow and mark your flick end point. The more you practise, the easier it becomes.
3. Keep some cotton buds and eye cream on hand to finetune the line as you go.
4. Line the lower waterline (inner lids) with black pencil.
5. Take the pencil into the lower lashline and join at the outer corner of the eye.
6. If you are happy with the shape, trace over the line with liquid liner — this adds intensity to the colour and makes it more long-wearing.
7. Curl lashes and apply two coats of mascara.
8. You can enhance the shape of the eye by adding individual lashes to the outer corner.
9. Contour the hollows of the cheeks and jawline using a brush and contouring powder.
10. Add a touch of luminizer to the cheekbones.
11. As a finishing touch, apply a little nude lipstick with your fingertips for just a hint of lip colour.

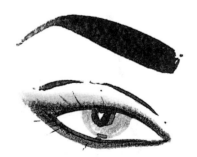 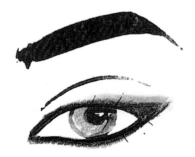

Tip

To soften the look, add a little eyeshadow.

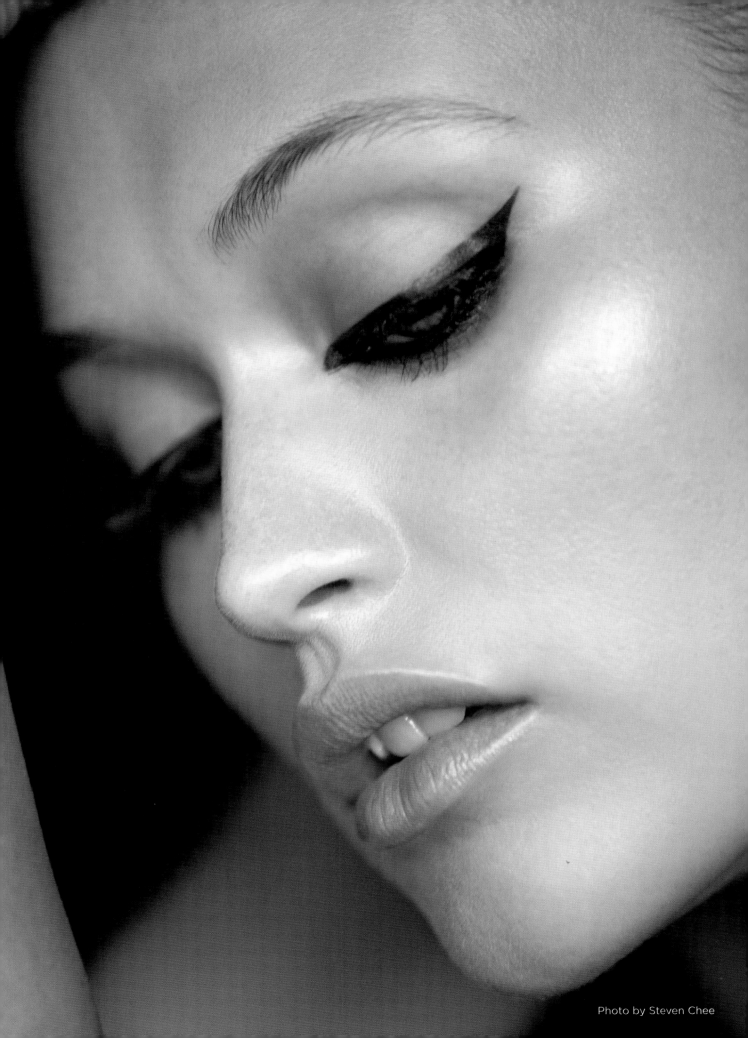

Photo by Steven Chee

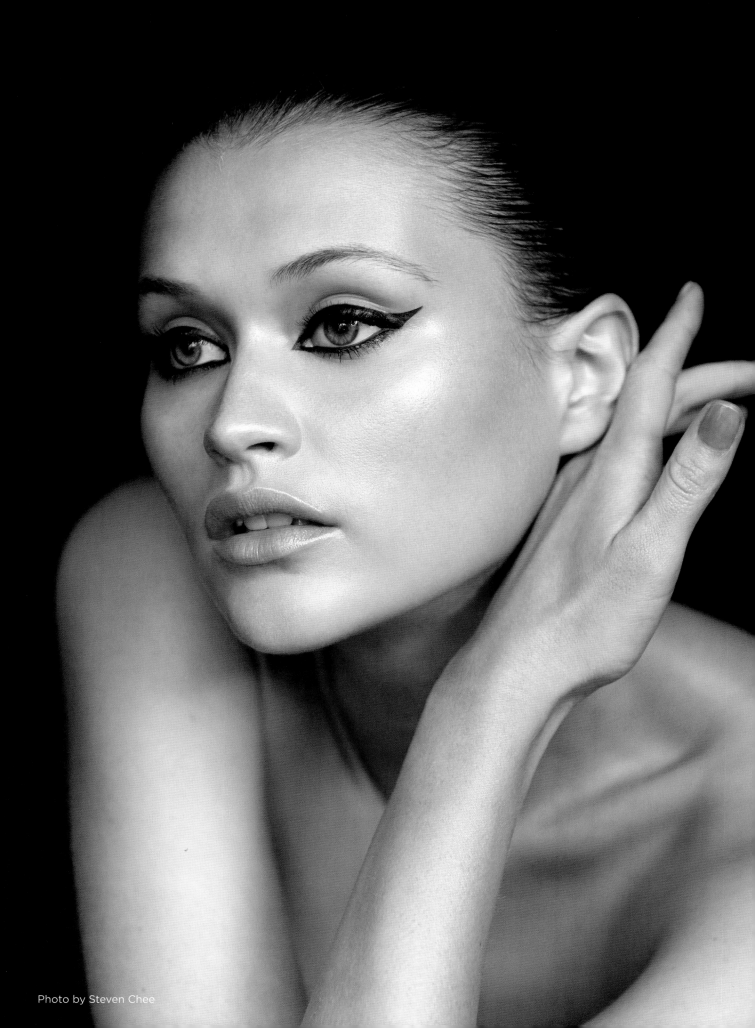

Photo by Steven Chee

The eye flick, part two

The eye flick can be pared down or taken to the max, depending on your mood. If you want to beef it up, here's how:

STEP BY STEP

1. Taking the original eye flick as your starting point, use a very sharp black liner to drag the point out further.

2. Balance it out by making the liner thicker along the upper lid and also thickening the flick.

3. Once you're happy with the shape, trace over with a liquid liner.

4. If necessary, add a little more bronzer to balance out the dominant eyes.

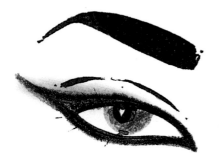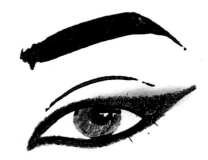

Beach-to-bar pink lips

This is a great summer lip look to take you from a day at the beach straight to sunset cocktails. It's fast and easy.

STEP BY STEP

1. To keep your face looking fresh, skip foundation and apply concealer sparingly to your trouble spots, such as the base of the nose and the chin.
2. If you've used waterproof mascara at the beginning of the day, it should still be in place.
3. Use luminizer on the high points of the face including the cheekbones and the bridge of the nose.
4. Chubby stick-pencil lipsticks are great for on-the-go application. There's no need for liner, just apply straight to the lips. Here, I've used a fuchsia pink.

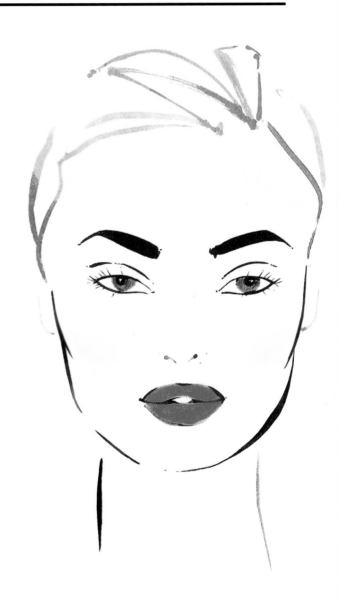

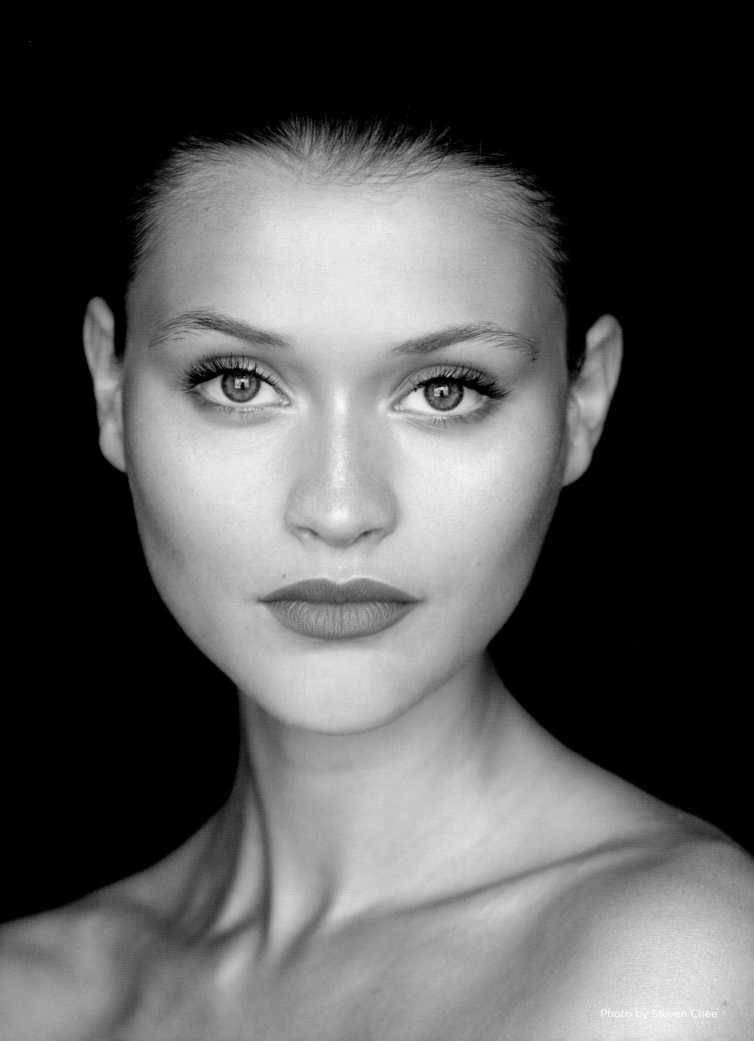

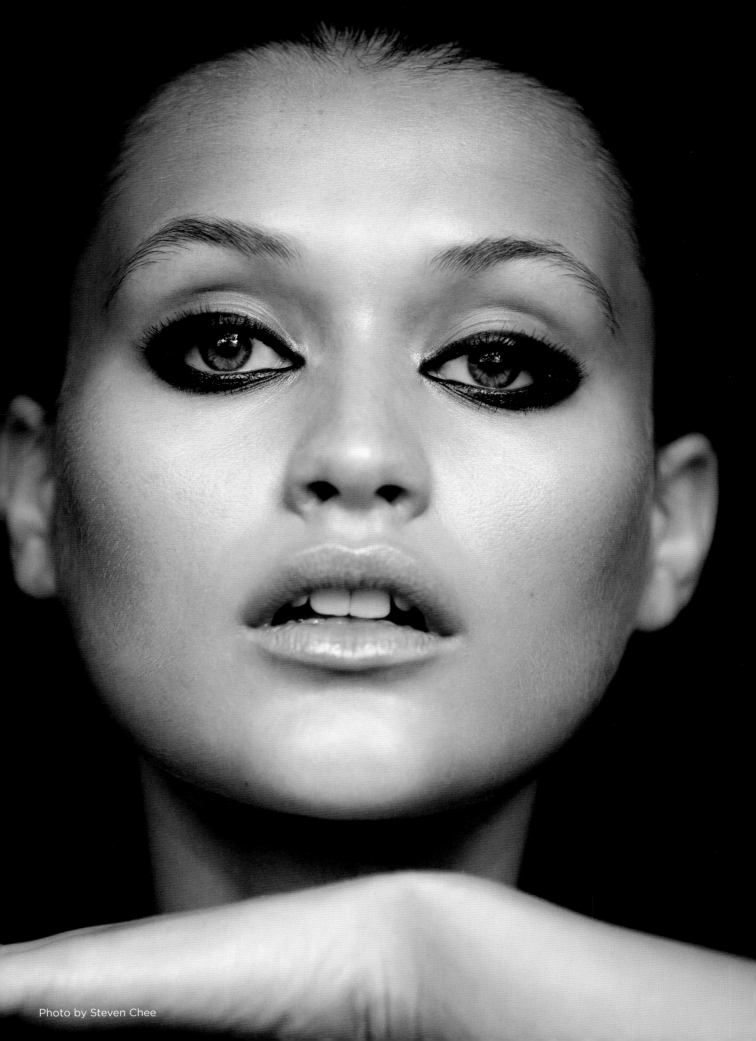

Photo by Steven Chee

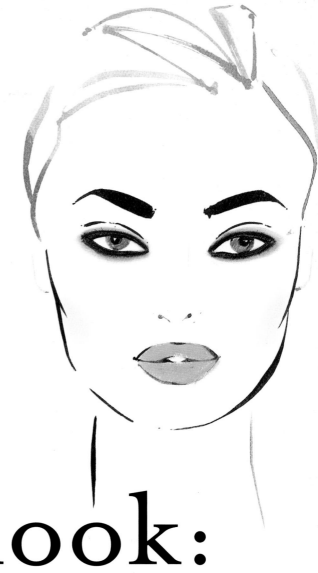

The It-girl look: Mary-Kate

The Olsen twins are the absolute 'It girls' of rock chic and their makeup look works for day or night. Let's look at Mary-Kate's makeup first. The key to this look is pairing natural-looking skin with a strong, 'lived-in' eye.

STEP BY STEP

1. Mix luminizer with your foundation to make it translucent. Alternatively, just conceal where necessary.
2. Curl your lashes.
3. Using a soft black kohl pencil, line the upper and lower waterline (inner lids).
4. Line the upper and lower lashline with a soft black kohl pencil. Smudge with a pointer brush.
5. Set with a little charcoal eyeshadow and press into the lashline. Use a cotton bud to smudge the edges. This gives a more 'lived-in' look.
6. Apply two coats of mascara.
7. Contour the cheek hollows.
8. Brush on cream bronzer to the perimeter of the face.
9. Last, but by no means least, apply your favourite beige-nude lip gloss.

The It-girl look: Ashley

This is a pared-down version of Mary-Kate's look — a little more rock and a little less kohl. Fresh-looking skin is key to this look.

STEP BY STEP

1. Mix some luminizer into your foundation to create a lighter base or just use concealer on the trouble spots.
2. Curl your lashes with a lash curler.
3. Using a soft brown kohl pencil, line the upper and lower waterline (inner lids) of your eyes.
4. Line the upper and lower lashline with a soft brown kohl pencil.
5. Draw the brown kohl into the base of your lashes and smudge with a pointer brush.
6. Press a little bronzer or brown shadow into the liner to set it. Use a cotton bud to smudge the edges to give it a more 'lived-in' look.
7. Contour the cheek hollows with a cream contour.
8. Apply bronzer with a brush to the perimeter of the face.
9. Groom brows with a brush.
10. Apply nude lipliner and lipstick.
11. For the finishing touch, dab a little translucent powder onto the centre of your lips with your finger.

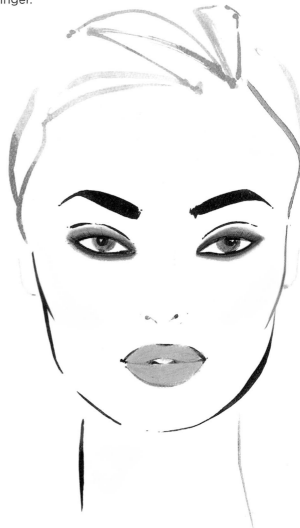

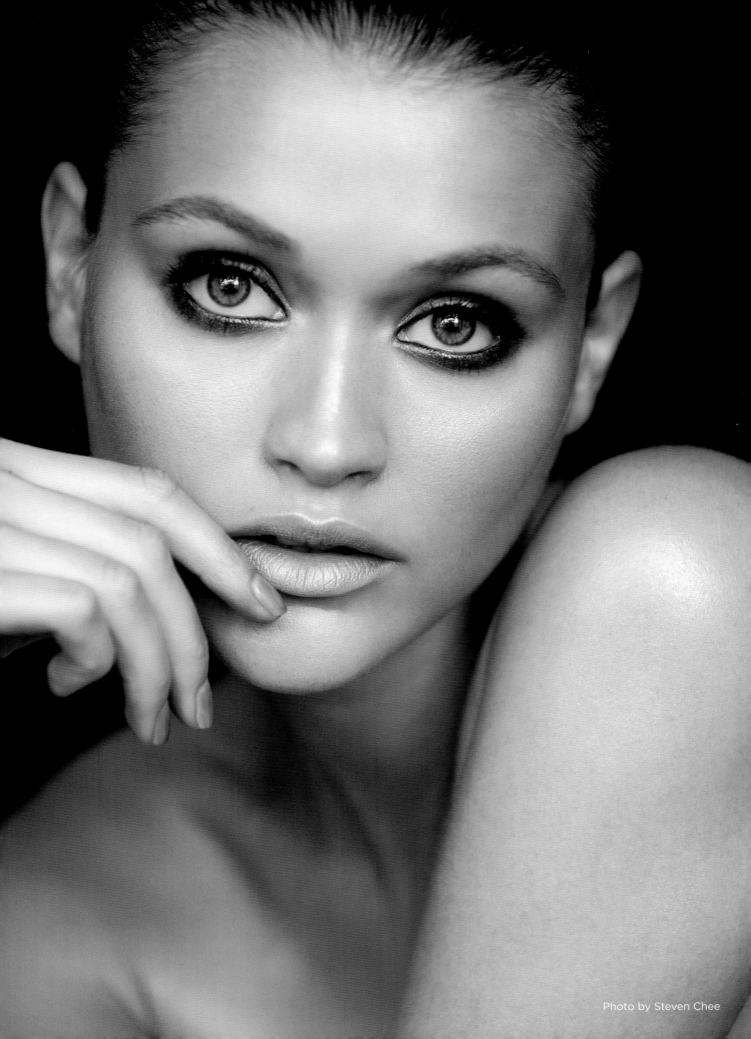

Photo by Steven Chee

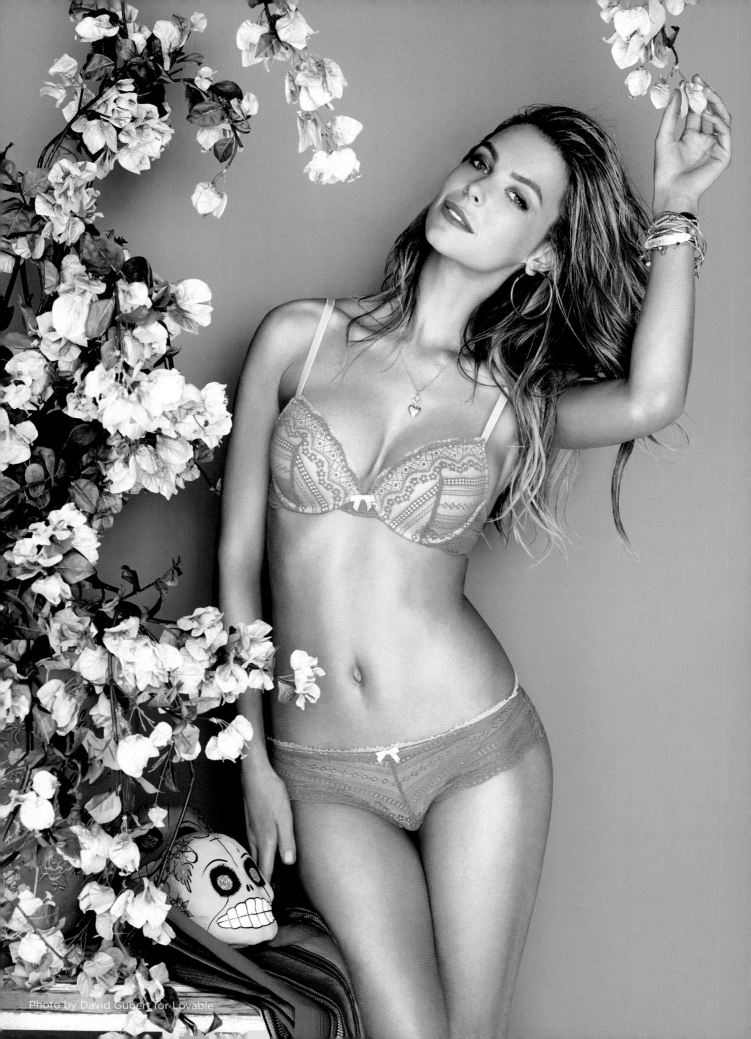

I believe in manicures.
I believe in over-
dressing. I believe in
primping at leisure
and wearing lipstick.
I believe in pink. I
believe happy girls are
the prettiest girls. I
believe that tomorrow
is another day, and …
I believe in miracles

— *AUDREY HEPBURN*

Transfo

mations

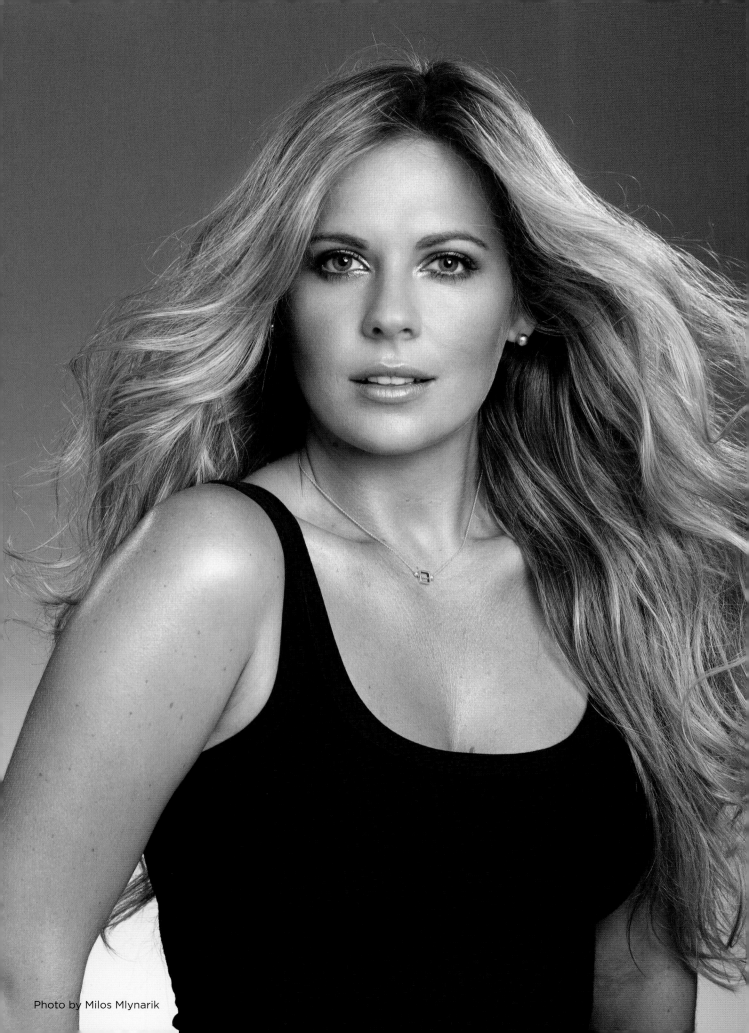

Photo by Milos Mlynarik

I'm constantly being asked for advice on makeup. From applying eyeliner to patchy foundation, the sort of things that drive us crazy about makeup are usually easy fixes. In this Transformations chapter, I wanted to take a cross-section of people in my life — from my daughter's teacher to mums I know from the playground — and show how easily these problems can be sorted.

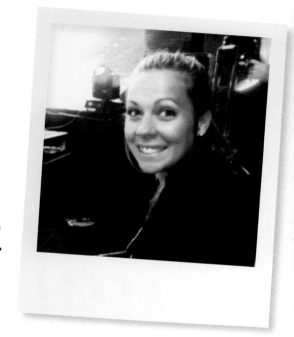

Rochelle

I first met Rochelle while we were both working with Geri Halliwell. We instantly bonded over eyeliner. Rochelle is a producer and works long weird hours and like most girls in their 20s she really wanted to master glowing skin with soft smoky eyes.

Problem

After a little investigation I realised Rochelle was making a very common mistake. She wanted natural-looking skin so she'd opted for tinted moisturiser. However, it wasn't giving her the cover she craved so she was applying too much. This is a girl who needs her foundation to last all day, and I'm afraid a tinted moisturiser just wasn't up for the job. Also Rochelle had light congestion under the skin (little white bumps). This is so easily fixed with the right exfoliant, so for Rochelle I suggested she use an exfoliant with glycolic acid.

On Rochelle I wanted to do the makeup I'm asked for most frequently: bronzed eye with dewy skin and a nude lip. It's a look that suits everyone and can be worn everywhere. This look is both classic and modern.

Solution

1. I applied a medium-brown cream eyeshadow to the lid and blended it with a brush into the crease.
2. Next I used a metallic bronze shadow to circle the lid and lower lashline.
3. I added a hint of gold shimmer to the inner corner of the eye.
4. I curled Rochelle's lashes and applied four coats of mascara.
5. I then applied an oil-free liquid matt foundation sparingly, starting at the centre of the face and blending out towards the hairline.
6. I added peachy cream blush to cheeks and blonde brow pencil to the brows.
7. I used a light, translucent loose powder on the T-zone to set the base.
8. Finally, I chose a nude pink lipstick, applied lightly to lips using the fingers.

Shelley

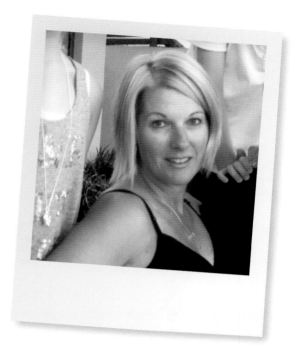

Problem

Shelley hated having her photo taken and found it impossible to smile during the process. She always looks great in my opinion, but she just wanted to tweak her look slightly to give herself a bit more confidence.

Solution

1. I mixed a little luminizer with a cream foundation and, starting at the centre of her face, worked out to the hairline.
2. I added a little concealer under her eyes.
3. Then I applied a light taupe cream shadow to the lid and blended it into the crease.
4. I used a blonde pencil for her brows.
5. As always, I applied cream bronzer with a brush to the perimeter of the face and the jawline.
6. I curled her lashes and followed with two coats of mascara, and then some individual lashes.
7. The finishing touch — satin-finish peach nude lipstick.

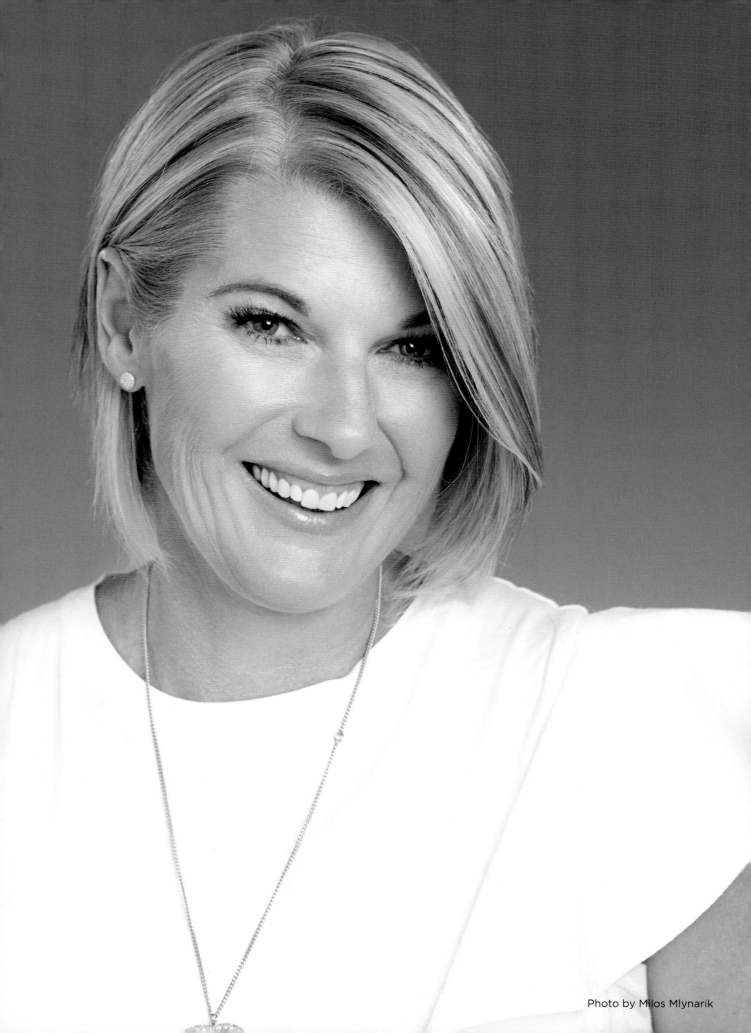

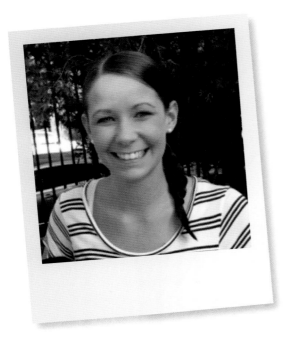

Miss Franko

Meet Miss Franko. She is my daughter's Year 1 teacher and the most beloved lady in the world. Miss Franko is a fantastic teacher with a warm personality and the patience of a saint. Her pupils adore her and when I asked my daughter why she loved Miss Franko so much, she replied, 'Because she's amazingly amazing.'

Problem

Miss Franko's brows were over-plucked. Also, her foundation was not an ideal match to her skin tone and had way more coverage than she needed. This gave the illusion she was trying to hide something, when in fact she has beautiful skin. First things first — I matched her foundation to her colouring by testing the shade along the jawline and onto her neck. Then I chose a more natural texture and coverage for her skin. I also wanted to experiment with some fun colour on her eyes to reflect her personality.

Solution

1. I prepped Miss Franko's skin and shaped her brows.
2. I then applied a light foundation all over her face to even out skin texture.
3. I used turquoise eyeliner and smudged it into the lower lashline, setting it using a matching powder eyeshadow.
4. Miss Franko needs to grow her brows, so I pencilled them in as much as possible. She's promised not to pluck them and we are going to move forward!
5. I added a light, pearl-gold, beige shadow to the lid to balance the vibrant colour underneath the eye and blended it into the crease using a blending brush.
6. I curled her lashes and applied two coats of mascara.
7. I then dusted peach cream blush to the apples of her cheeks and lightly contoured for a little extra definition.
8. And the finishing touch — a natural gloss.

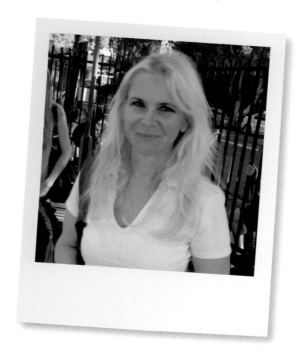

Lana

Problem

Lana is addicted to black eyeliner but wanted to find out how to make it last all day. I wanted to introduce her to long-wear makeup and also soften her skin tone to balance out her dark eyes.

Solution

1. To create Lana's signature liner, I used a long-wear eye pencil to create the line and then sealed it using a liquid liner.
2. I added lashings and lashings of mascara.
3. I massaged an illuminating moisturiser into Lana's skin, followed by a light liquid foundation, and applied concealer sparingly.
4. I added a cream bronzer to lift her complexion.
5. I then applied luminizer to the high points of the face.
6. A soft pink gloss completes the look.

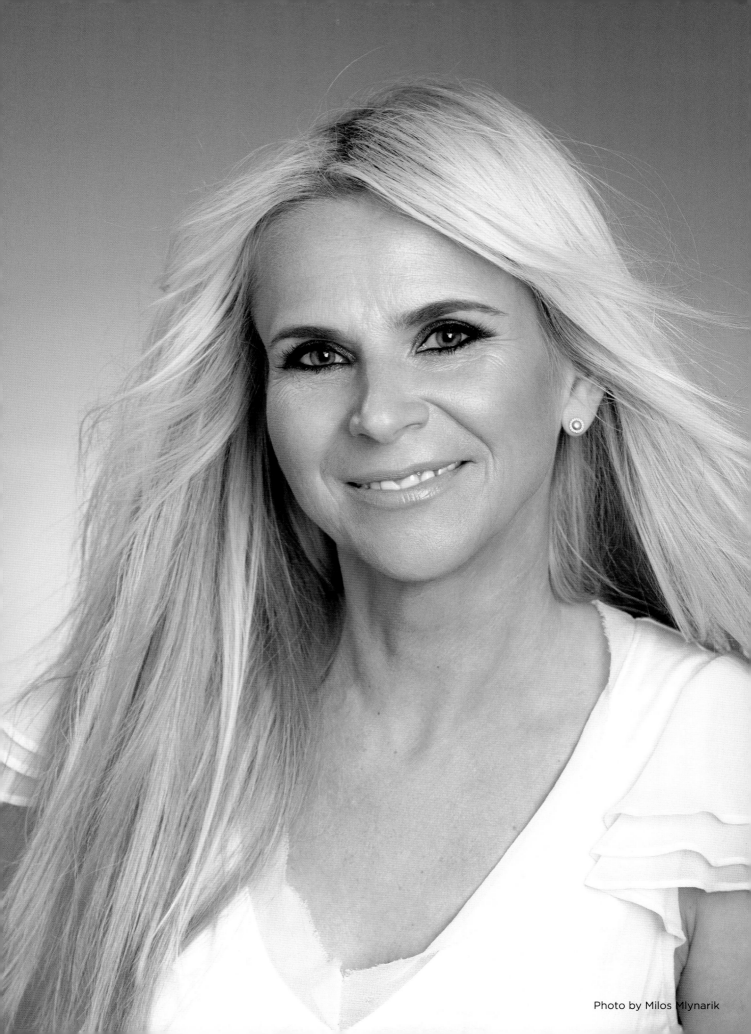

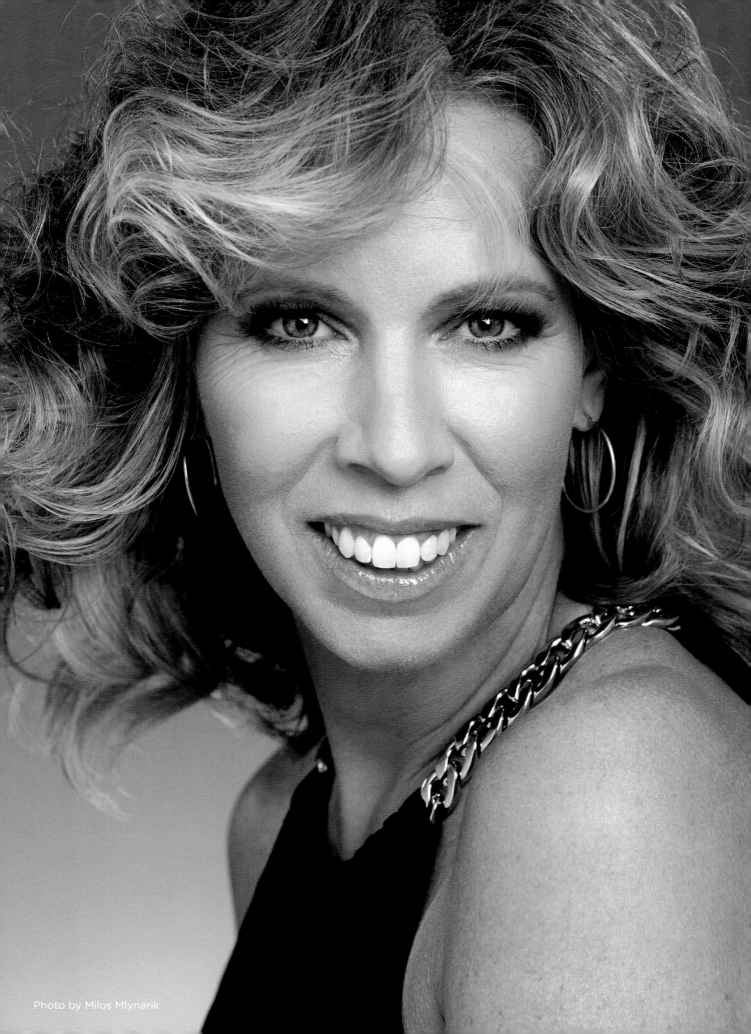

Jacinta

Problem

Jacinta had trouble making her foundation last the distance. The first thing to address was to recommend a good exfoliation routine. The next was to apply a high-quality matt foundation as well as some strategic contouring.

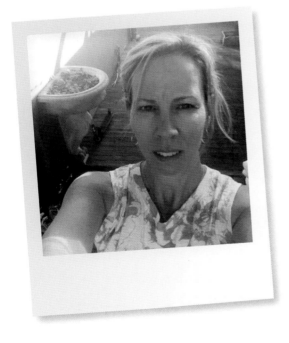

Solution

1. I started by using a thermal exfoliator.
2. I applied a mask to plump up the skin.
3. I asked Jacinta to suck in her cheeks and used a cream contour on her cheeks and jawline.
4. Soft coral cream blush, worn high on the apples of her cheeks, gives the illusion of strong cheekbones. I also added a touch of highlighter.
5. I bronzed up Jacinta's eyes by applying bronze shadow to the upper and lower lashline.
6. I also added some individual lashes.
7. I finished with a light dusting of bronzing powder and a slick of nude gloss for her lips.

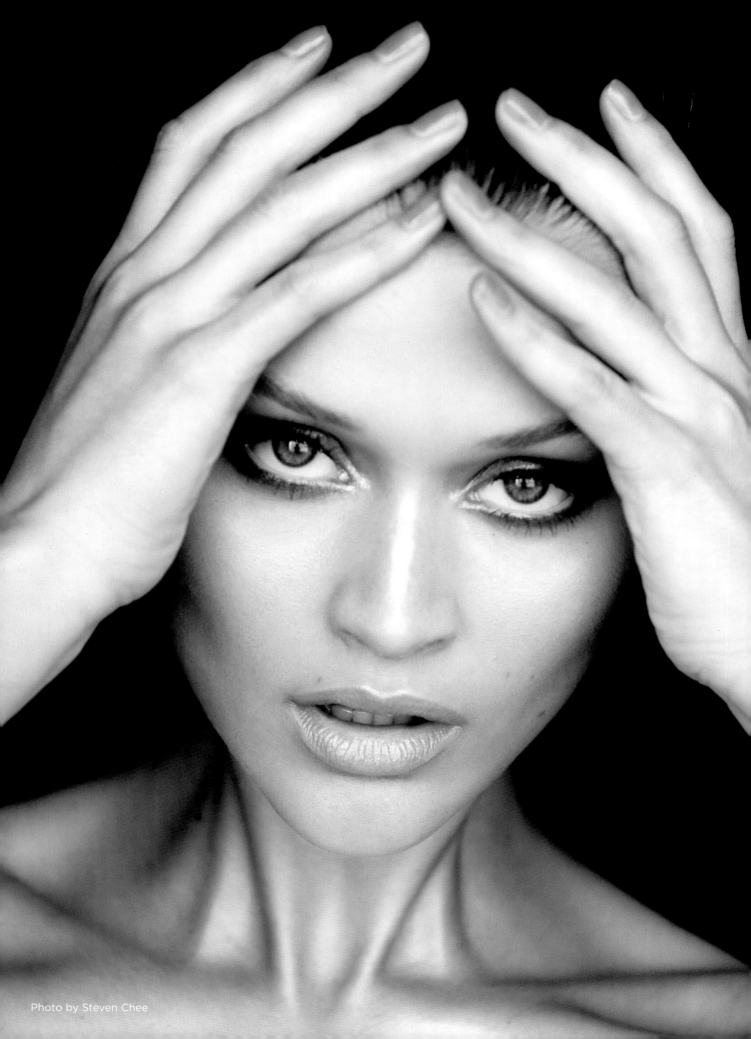

Look at me, a big old black man under all of this makeup and if I can look beautiful, so can you

— RUPAUL

Anna

Problem

Anna doesn't really wear much makeup and has her hair tied up most of the time. I wanted to show her a few basic makeup tips and she wanted to know how to use concealer.

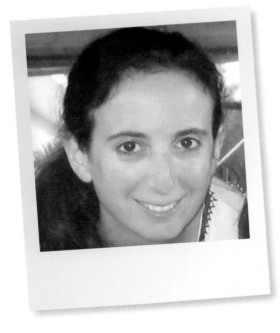

Solution

1. I prepped Anna's skin with a good moisturiser.
2. Next I applied a light cream foundation to the centre of her face and worked it out to the hairline.
3. I followed this with a concealer where needed, particularly under the eyes.
4. I smudged a deep plum shadow into Anna's lashline and curled her lashes, finishing with two coats of mascara.
5. I then applied cream blush to the cheeks and lips.
6. I dusted a translucent powder on her T-zone and groomed her brows.

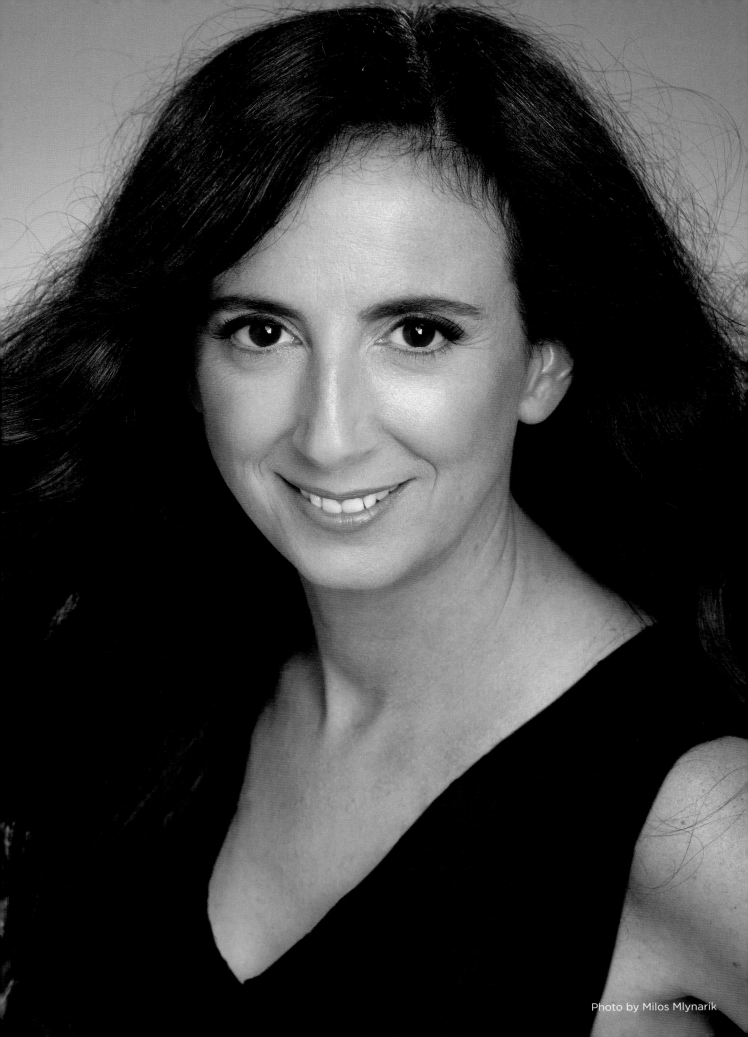

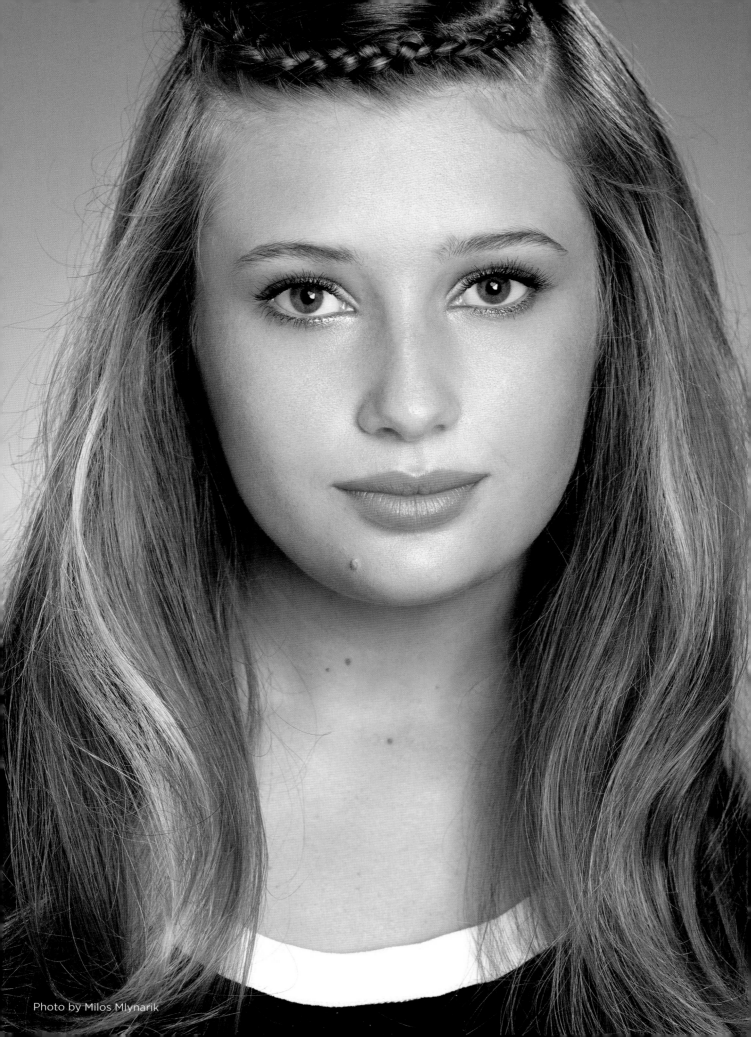

Photo by Milos Mlynarik

Ruby

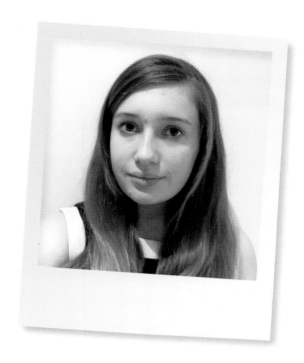

Ruby's mum, Pamela, and I are friends and colleagues. I adore Pamela, so of course when she asked me if her fifteen-year-old daughter could do some work experience with me, I was more than happy to oblige. Little did Pamela know the Pandora's Box she was opening for Ruby! After just one day of shooting with me, Ruby caught the makeup bug big time. Since then, Ruby has come to work with me on school holidays and weekends. I love having her as part of the team and observing her confidence with makeup grow and grow.

Problem

For the shot, I wanted to create an age-appropriate makeup for Ruby. At this age, makeup should be used as an accessory, never as a mask. Many teenagers needlessly apply heavy foundations, without realising the potential of their naturally glowing young skin. The best advice I can give girls of this age is to take care of your skin and, above all, cleanse really well before bed — then it becomes second nature.

For Ruby, I went for soft, pretty makeup — with a 'kick-ass' lip.

Solution

1. I started with a very sheer foundation and a little concealer where needed.
2. Next I curled Ruby's lashes and applied pearl-gold, beige eyeshadow to the lid and lightly on the lower lashline.
3. I added bronzer with a brush to the perimeter of Ruby's face and luminizer to her cheekbones.
4. I finished with a pretty pink lipstick pencil.

Jamie

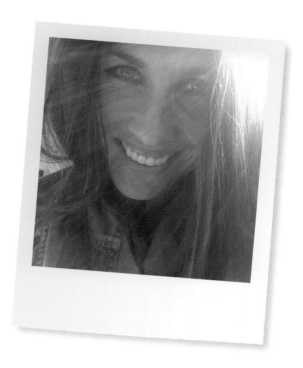

Jamie is the designer and owner of One Teaspoon. She is also one of the most amazing women I have ever been blessed to have in my life. She's a great mum, a power businesswoman and the queen of multitasking, all while being uber cool, 100% genuine, friendly and with a fabulous sense of humour.

Problem

Jamie just had a little girl a couple of months before shooting this photo, and being the wonder woman she is, she breastfeeds while taking care of her two little boys and running her empire. Not surprisingly, her skin is a little dehydrated and is quick to lose its glow.

First I did an intensive moisturising eye mask and face mask, leaving it on for twenty minutes. Then I spent ten minutes massaging a rich moisturiser into her skin. Before applying foundation, I applied a cream luminizer to her whole face, about which she said, 'What was that?!' So the treatment and the luminizer sorted out Jamie's skin issue, but just for fun I really wanted to smoke up her eyes.

Pregnancy, childbirth and breastfeeding can take a real toll on your skin. One minute your skin is dry, the next it's oily. After I had my daughter, my skin suffered as well. The main thing is not to panic, and remember it will only be temporary. Don't over treat these problems, as they're mostly hormone related. Just keep exfoliating to remove any extra dry skin you have, moisturise and drink water, and you'll soon be back to normal.

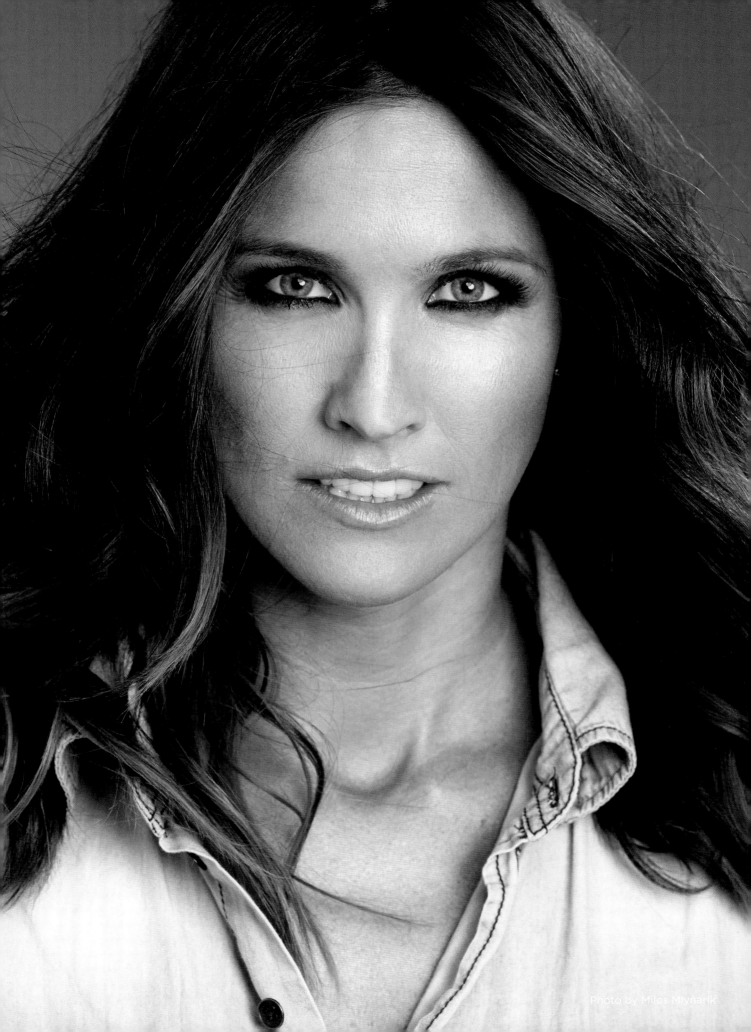

Solution

1. I applied foundation and a liquid luminizer to Jamie's face, adding a touch of translucent powder to the T-zone.

2. I used a grey cream eyeshadow on her lids and blended it into the crease with a blending brush.

3. I added black liner to Jamie's upper and lower waterline for impact as well as into the upper and lower lashline, which I then smudged with a pointer brush.

4. I applied dark grey shadow to the lashline, smudging it into the liner.

5. I added more smoke to the lids with dark grey shadow applied with a shadow brush.

6. I curled her lashes and applied thickening black mascara.

7. Medium-brown pencil added definition to Jamie's brows.

8. I then added more luminizer to the cheekbones and the bridge of the nose, followed by a light application of cream bronzer to frame the face.

9. I slicked on the essential nude lipstick, one that matched her skin tone, and finished with a dab of powder in the centre of the lips.

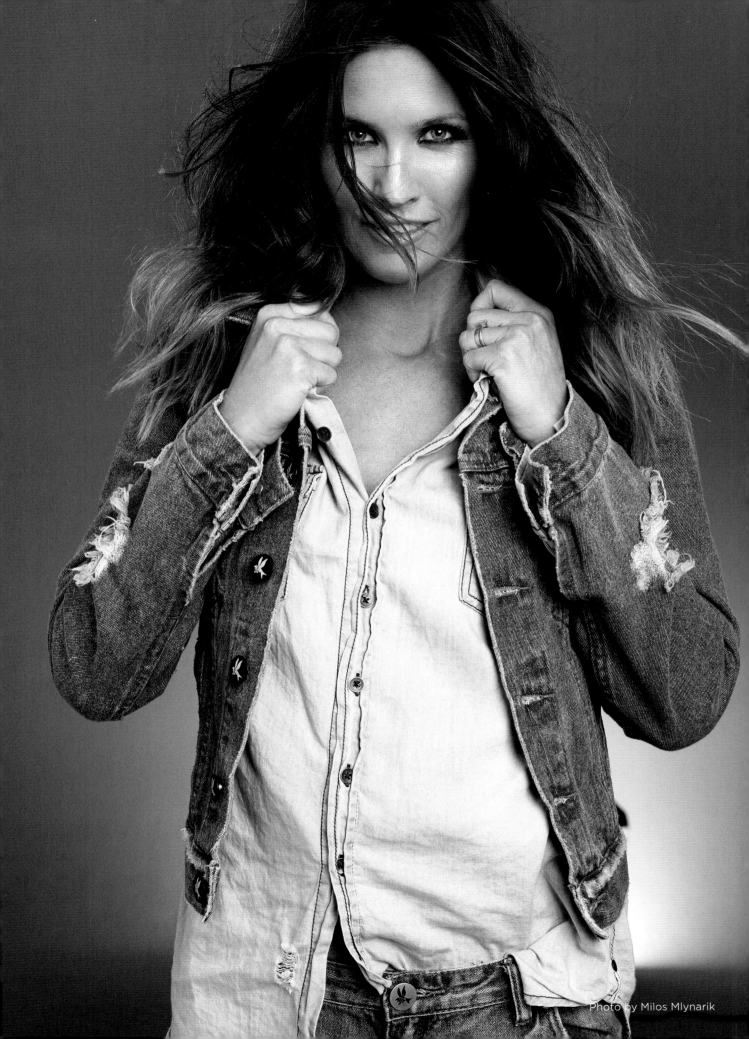

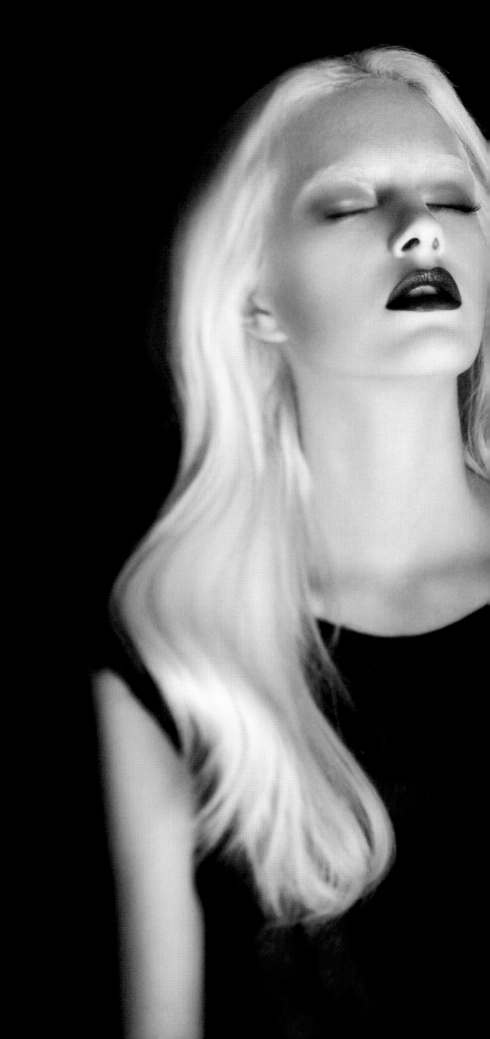

Photo by Liz Ham

The secret of staying young is to live honestly, eat slowly and lie about your age

— *LUCILLE BALL*

Behind

the Scenes

Georges Antoni
for Harper's Bazaar

This was shot on location at the iconic Tamarama Beach, with my beautiful girl Jennifer Hawkins looking stunning. As so often happens when you shoot at the beach, she ended up in the water, so I used long-wear makeup for this shoot and kept powder to a minimum for a more luminous look.

Tip

A hint of foundation and a dash of luminizer mixed with sunscreen makes great body makeup.

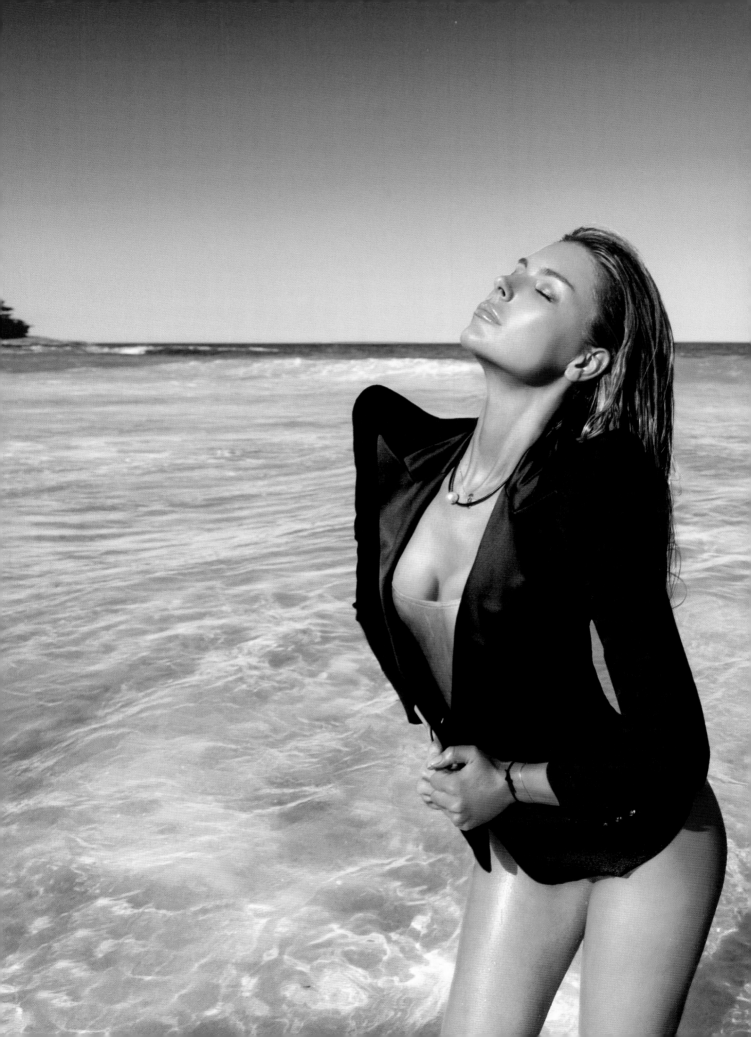

Sam Haskins
for Harper's Bazaar

I am so honoured and fortunate to have had the experience of working with renowned and now sadly deceased Sam Haskins. He is a true legend, known chiefly for his infamous work, *Cowboy Kate*. For this look I wanted to give the model's brows a lot more definition, so I chose a brow pencil in a lighter colour than her natural brow to lend some old-world Hollywood glamour.

Tip

A well-groomed brow not only gives a more youthful appearance, it also gives definition to your face and jawline.

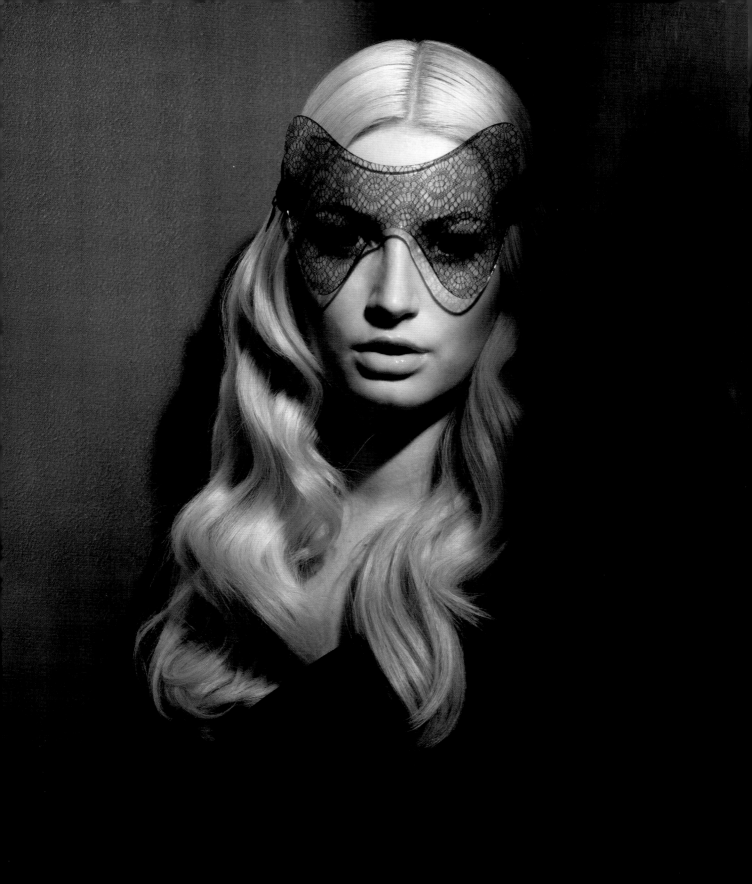

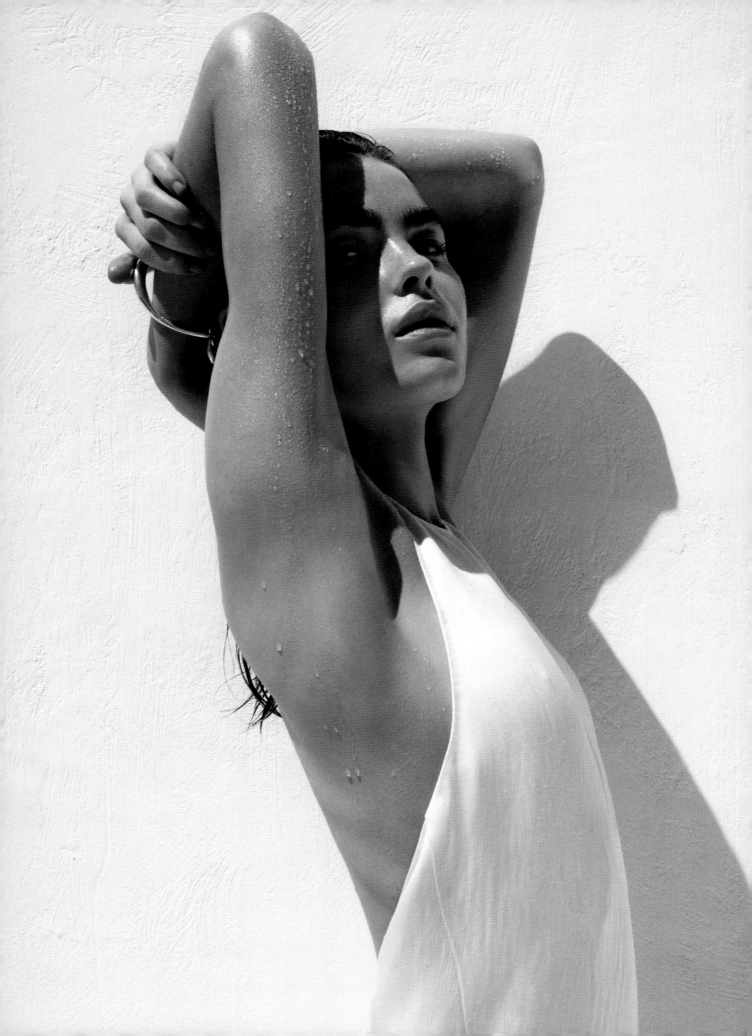

Pierre Toussaint
for Harper's Bazaar

This was a shoot for *Harper's Bazaar,* featuring the incredible Bambi. My talented friend Pierre Toussaint shot it at Icebergs at Bondi Beach in Sydney. The brief was all-white clothes with a no-makeup, sun-kissed, wet look. The challenge here was to tan up Bambi's skin without losing the effortlessly fresh feel. I also needed something waterproof because her skin would be wet and the clothes were white. I opted for a bronzing body gel — it dries instantly, doesn't come off on clothes, has zero sparkle and washes off easily after a shoot. For Bambi's face, I kept it really simple — just luminizer, concealer, tinted lip balm and a little definition to the eyes.

Tip

Always remember your sunscreen, even with a no-makeup look. Make sure it has both UVA and UVB protection.

Nick Leary for Linneys Collection

This campaign was shot on what felt like the coldest day ever in New South Wales. As Murphy's Law dictates, the models — Jessica van der Steen and David Genat — were wearing next to nothing bar the exquisite Linneys jewellery collection. When my manager first saw these shots, she declared that this was the makeup she wanted for her wedding. The look is sophisticated, with definition given to the eyes using neutral tones and individual lashes. As a result of the cold conditions, however, my main challenge was fighting off goosebumps and covering up a red nose. Like the true professionals they are, Jessica and David had warmth in their eyes in every shot, despite the freezing conditions.

Tip

Add cream highlighter to the inner corner of the eyes to open them up.

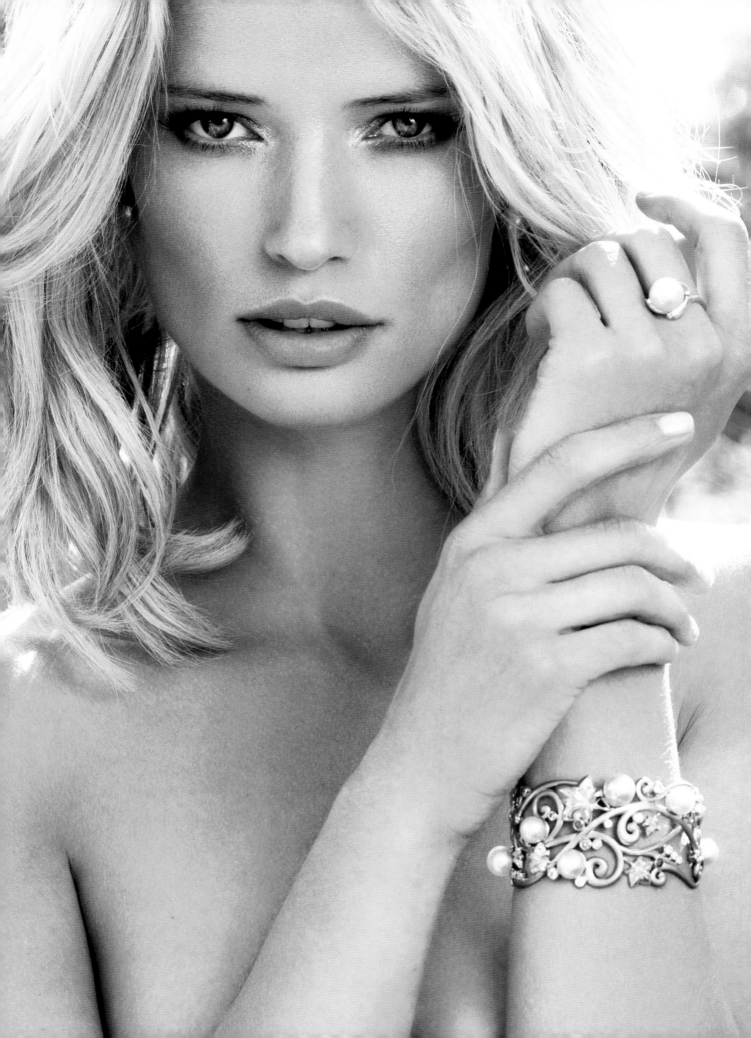

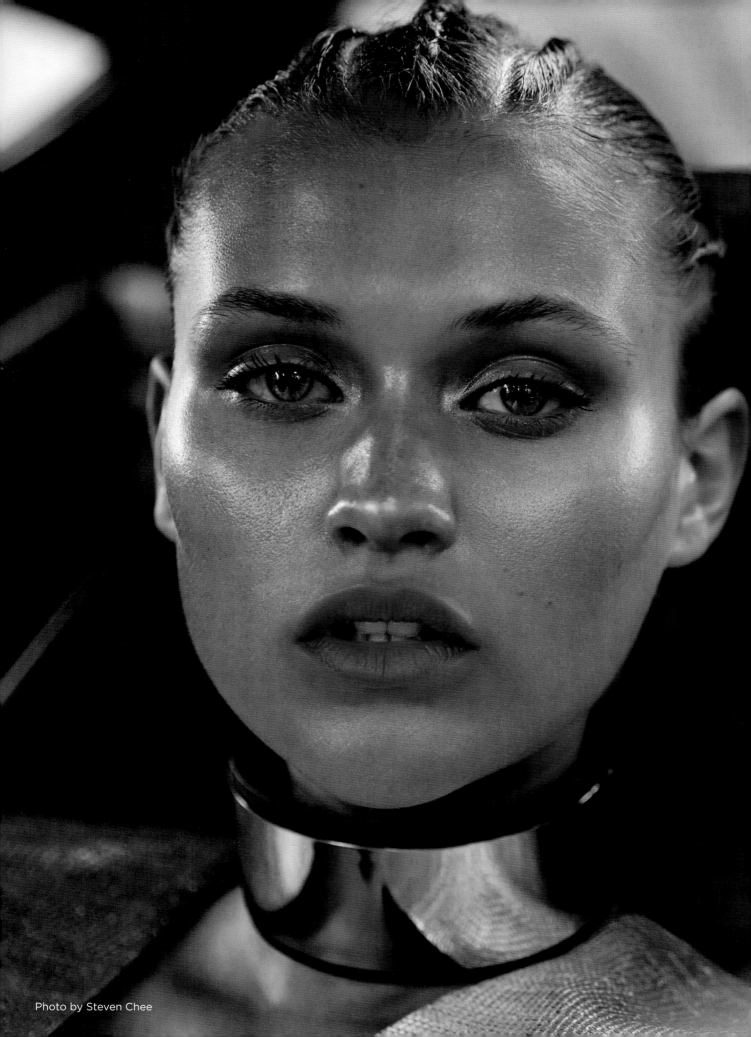

Photo by Steven Chee

You are
not born
glamorous,
glamour is
created

— *MAX FACTOR*

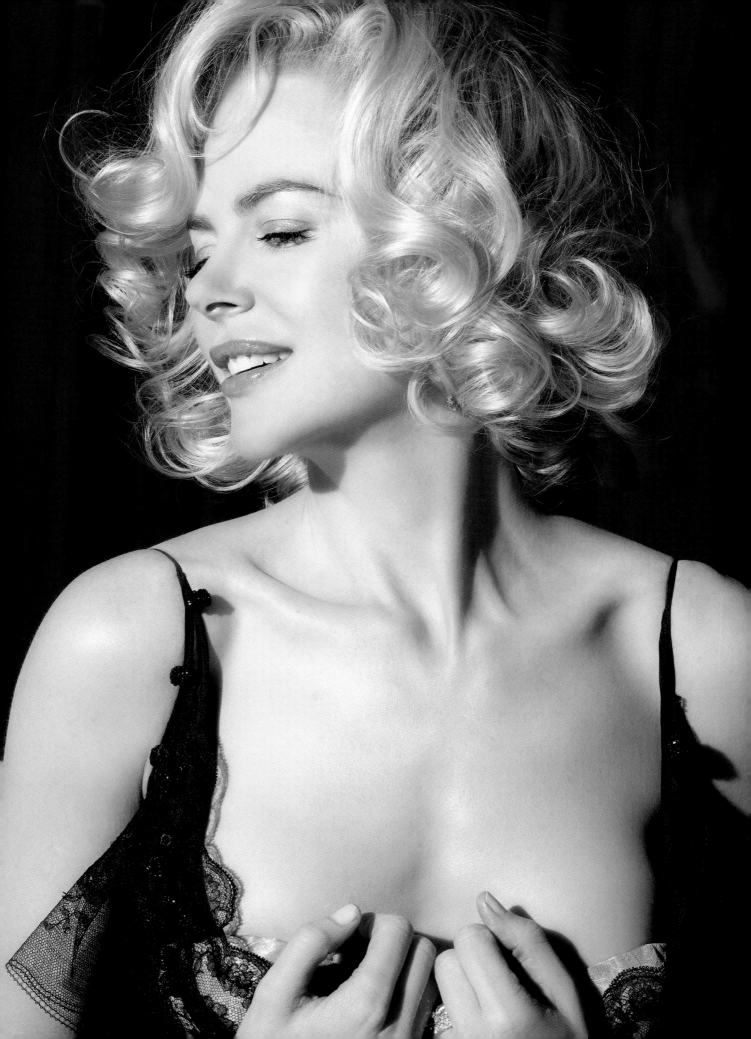

Alan Gelati
for Harper's Bazaar

This would have to be one of my all-time favourite shoots — Nicole Kidman for *Harper's Bazaar*.
It was an ode to Marilyn Monroe, so I kept the makeup natural to show off Nicole's amazing skin and added a hint of a 1950s Monroesque brow.

Steven Chee
for Vogue

This was shot on location in Sydney for a *Vogue* cover story featuring Cate Blanchett, with the always-incredible Steven Chee and my wonderful, talented, warm-hearted friend Renya Xydis on hair. We wanted to give beautiful Cate a sun-kissed glow, so it was important to keep everything else fresh.

Tip

For very fair skin, use cream bronzer on the face. Apply sparingly and blend well. For a more intense bronze, layer up and always check your blending in good light.

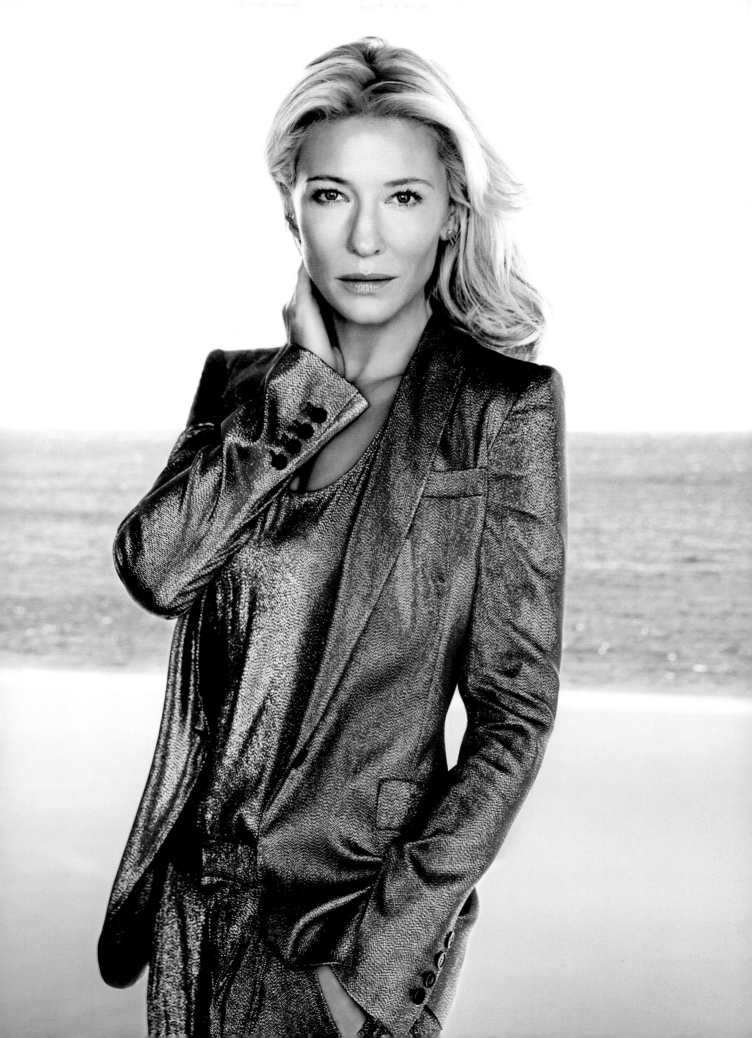

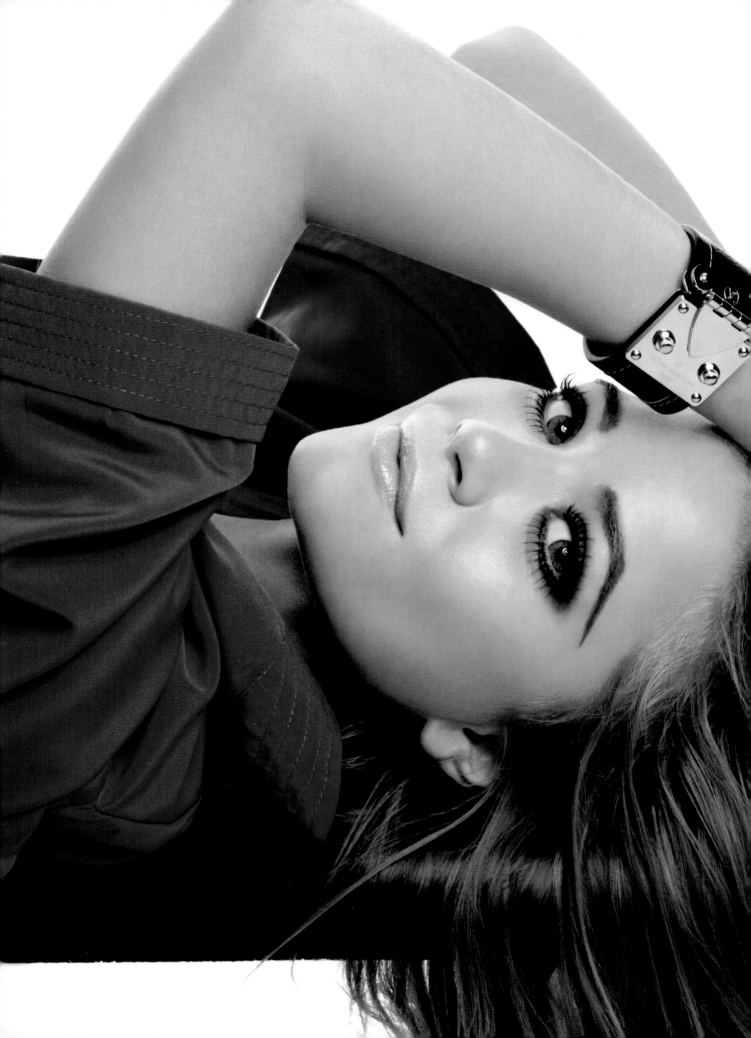

Daniel Smith
for Harper's Bazaar

This was the inside shot of a cover shoot I did with Mary-Kate Olsen for *Harper's Bazaar*, photographed by Daniel Smith. We wanted a 1960s vibe, so I used strip lashes on both upper and lower lashes. A nude lipstick, similar to Mary-Kate's skin tone, added to the overall feel.

Tip

When using false lashes, allow the glue to go tacky before applying.

Pierre Toussaint *for Kailis*

With the brilliant Pierre Toussaint behind the lens, and fellow Irish and funny man Michael Brennan on hair. They made it such an enjoyable day. Natalie Imbruglia has the most gorgeous face, and I really wanted her natural beauty to shine through, so I kept the makeup to a bare minimum and just used some mascara and a tinted lip conditioner.

Tip

Dare to bare now and again — sometimes all you need is concealer.

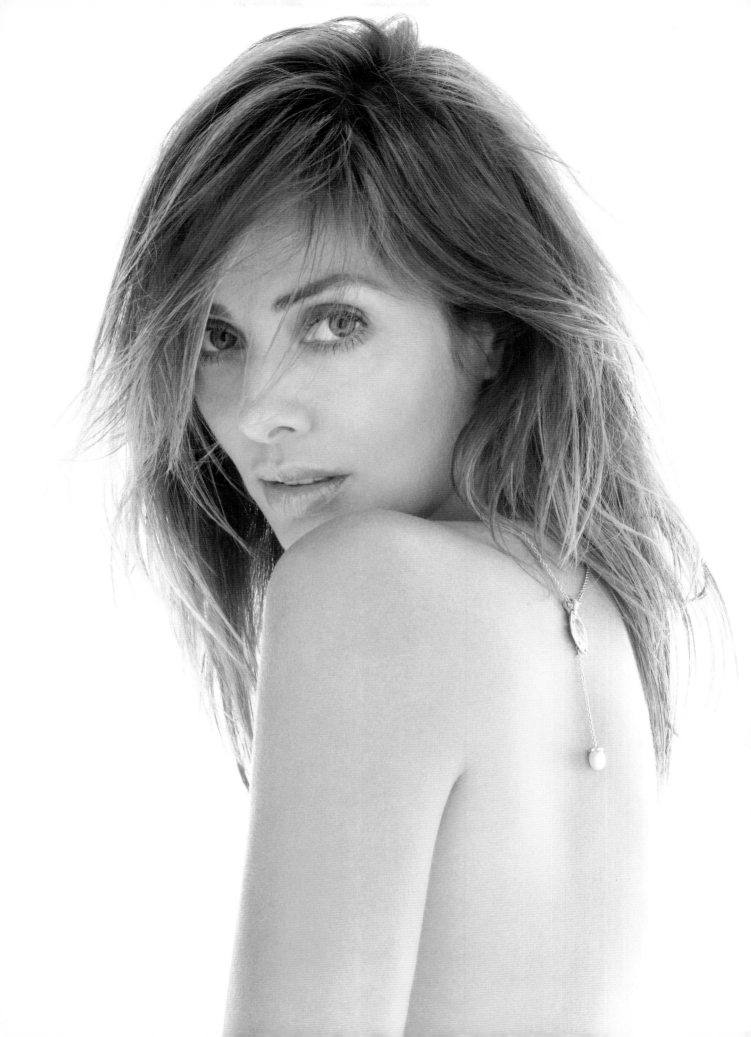

Polish

ur Look

Working with colour

It's a question I'm asked time and time again: 'What colour best suits my eyes?' Before I answer, let's go back to the fundamentals. The key to emphasising your eyes is working with your eye shape rather than with their colour. It's amazing how some strategically placed eyeliner can give you an instant eyelift or a pop of shimmer highlighter can open up close-set eyes. So, now on to answer the colour question — it's all to do with Sir Isaac Newton's colour wheel.

Colours are derived from various combinations of red, yellow or blue, also known as the primary colours (see colour wheel opposite). Secondary colours are made by mixing two primary colours together to form the secondary colour: red and blue make purple; blue and yellow create green; and red and yellow make orange. Mixing one primary and one secondary colour together creates a tertiary colour.

Colours that sit opposite each other on the colour wheel are called complementary colours and when placed side by side they will appear stronger. Choosing an eyeshadow that is on the opposite side of the colour wheel to your eye colour will make your eye colour 'pop'. It's important to carefully consider the colours you choose for your eyeshadow because they also need to work with your skin tone and the rest of your makeup.

My take on colour is much more free-form. I think you should play around with lots of colours — the sky's the limit!

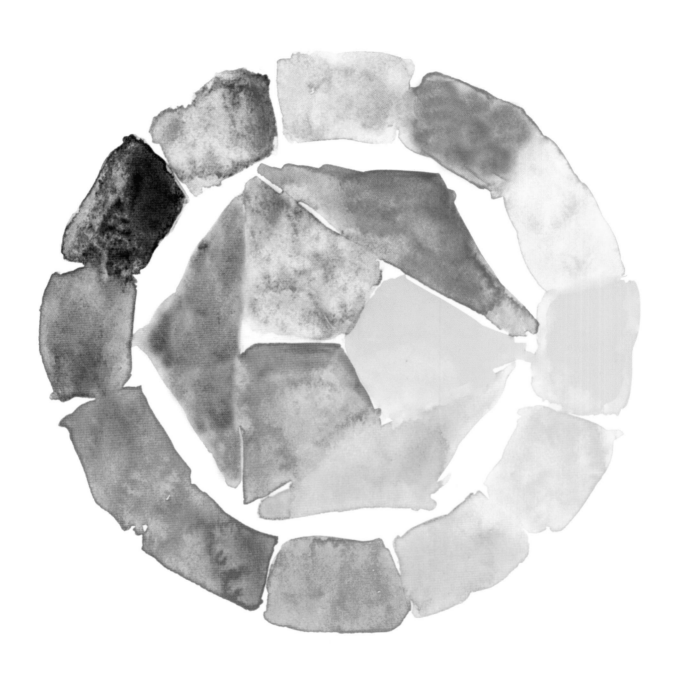

The key to successful self-tanning

First things first — if you're going to fake tan, always use a tanning mitt; it will change your life. It speeds up the process, making blending a breeze — and no more orange palms!

There's a vast array of self-tanners on the market, including ones that are applied and then develop over four to six hours; gradual tanners that are applied daily to develop a soft golden glow; and wash-off body bronzers. Self-tanners come as creams (good for dry skin); mousses (quick-drying and applied with a mitt); and aerosol sprays (great for tricky areas including hands and back).

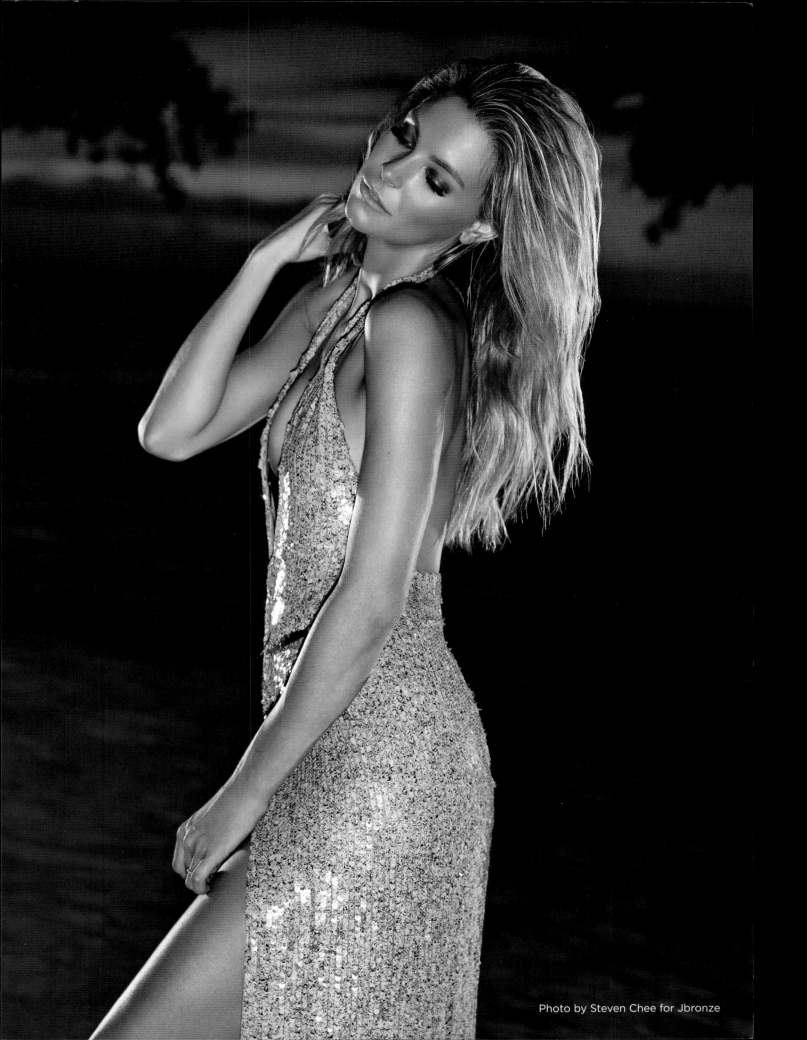

Photo by Steven Chee for Jbronze

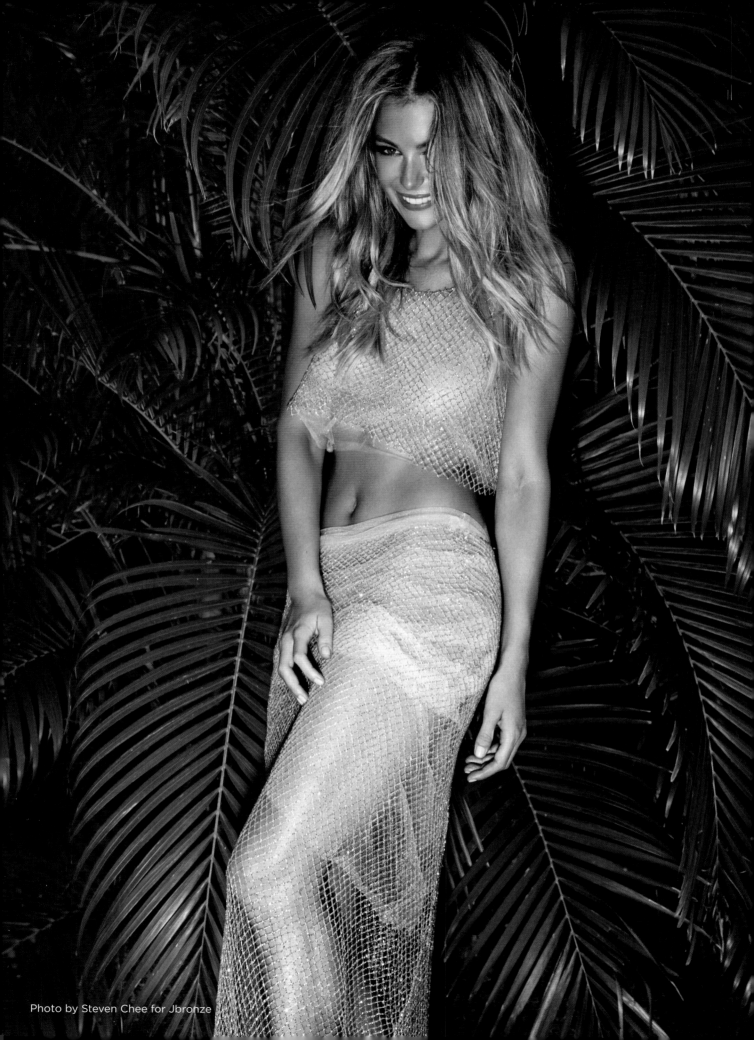

Photo by Steven Chee for Jbronze

Application

Thorough preparation is the key to avoiding patchy application. Make sure you exfoliate your skin before applying the tanning product. Use moisturiser in any areas that are likely to 'grab' the tan, for example the brows, elbows, heels, cuticles and the back of the wrists. Then, using a tanning mitt, work in a liberal amount of fake tan, starting at the feet and working upwards. Allow the tan to cure for four to six hours before showering or wearing tight clothes.

Troubleshooting

- Exfoliate often between tans and never ever apply tan over an already patchy one — it will only make it worse.
- Don't wear deodorant or fragrance while tanning — it can turn the tan green.
- Remove stains using baking soda and water.
- Remember, a fake tan does not protect you from the sun, so it's essential to wear sunscreen.
- If you need to wax or shave, do so at least a day before tanning.

Tip

Be careful with self-tanners. Don't let them build up on your face because they can block your pores.

Body makeup

Nothing puts the ultimate polish on your look like a little body makeup. It can be used to reflect the texture, feel and look of any makeup. My favourite technique is to apply a very sheer body makeup to the arms and legs and then add a little luminizer to the ball of the shoulder and down the centre of the legs. Make sure you conceal any scars or bruises with concealer.

For daywear, choose a rich body moisturiser to give your skin a glowing radiance. Body shimmer powder also looks fantastic. And remember — if you've gone for a sun-kissed glow on your face, you should take that onto your body as well. Apply a self-tan the night before, or a wash-off tan on the day.

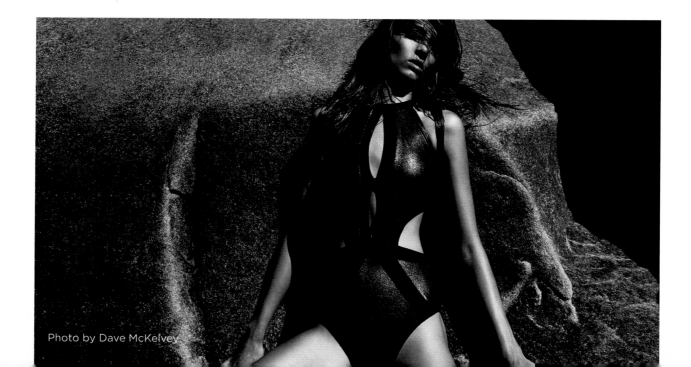

Photo by Dave McKelvey

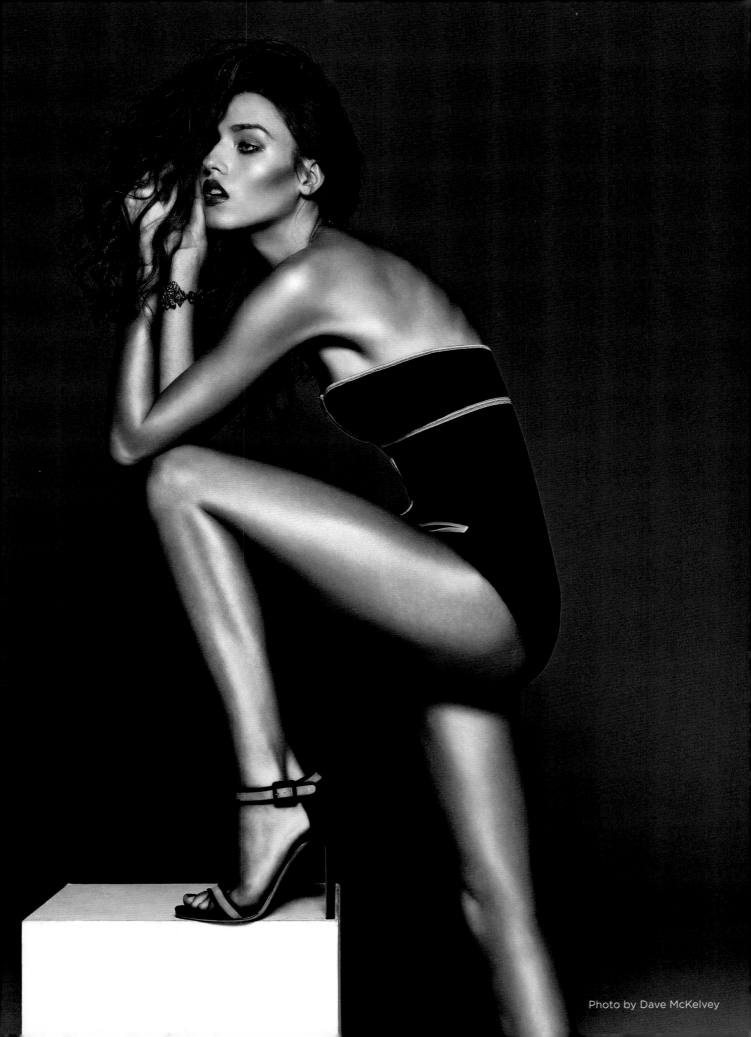

Photo by Dave McKelvey

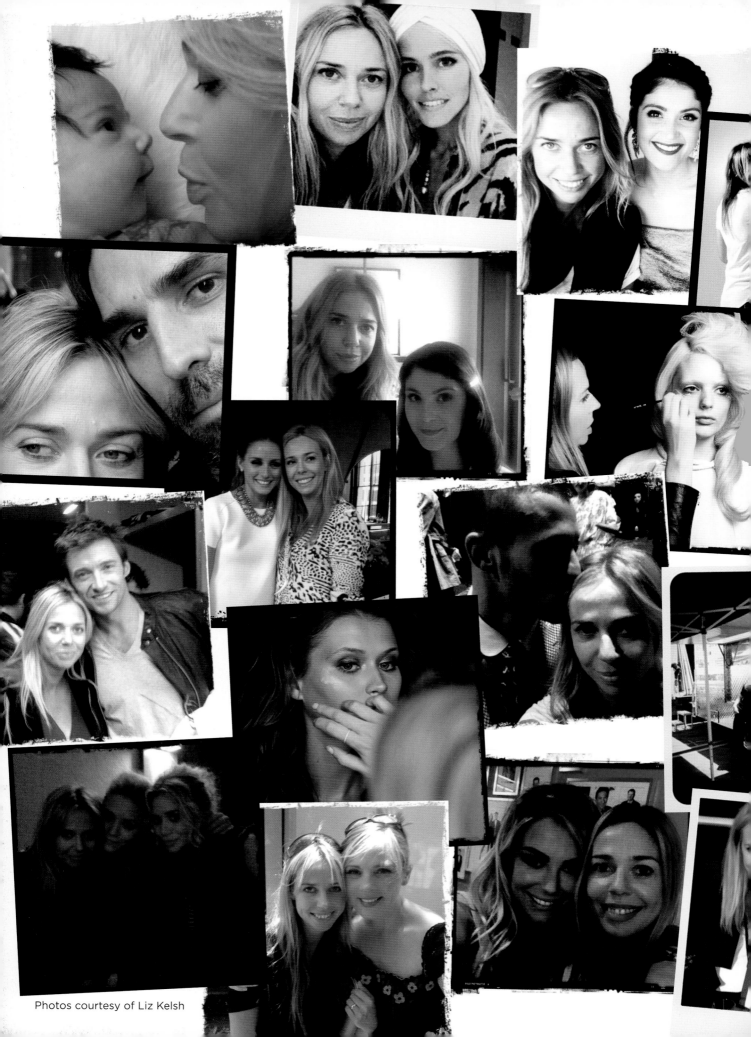

Photos courtesy of Liz Kelsh

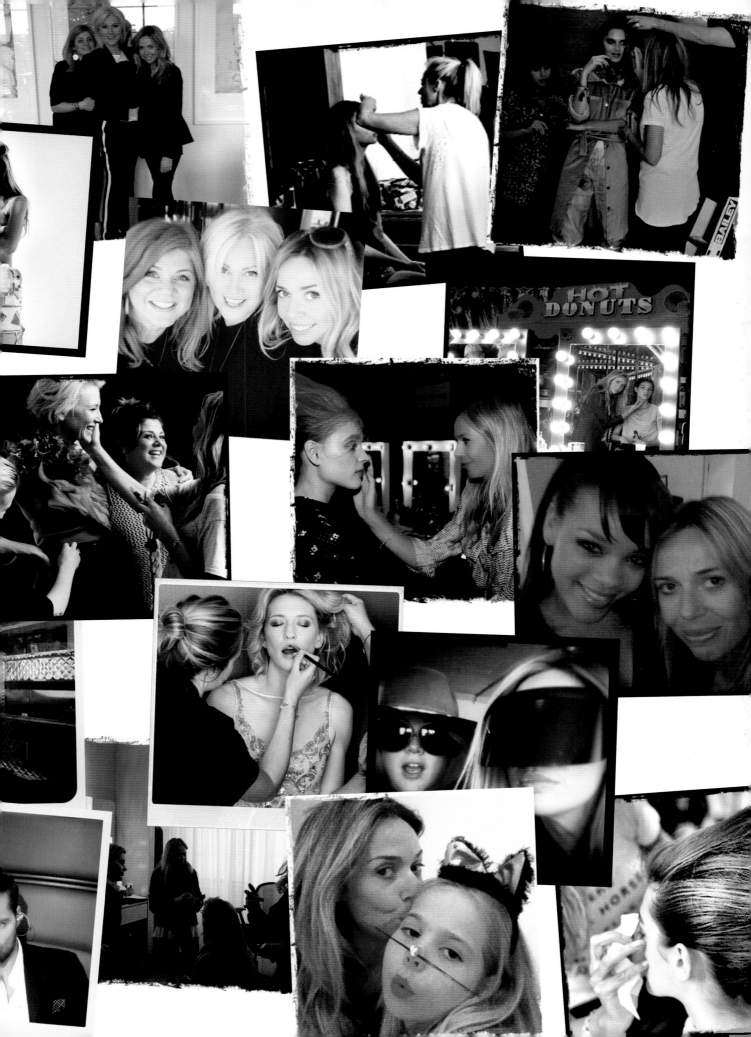

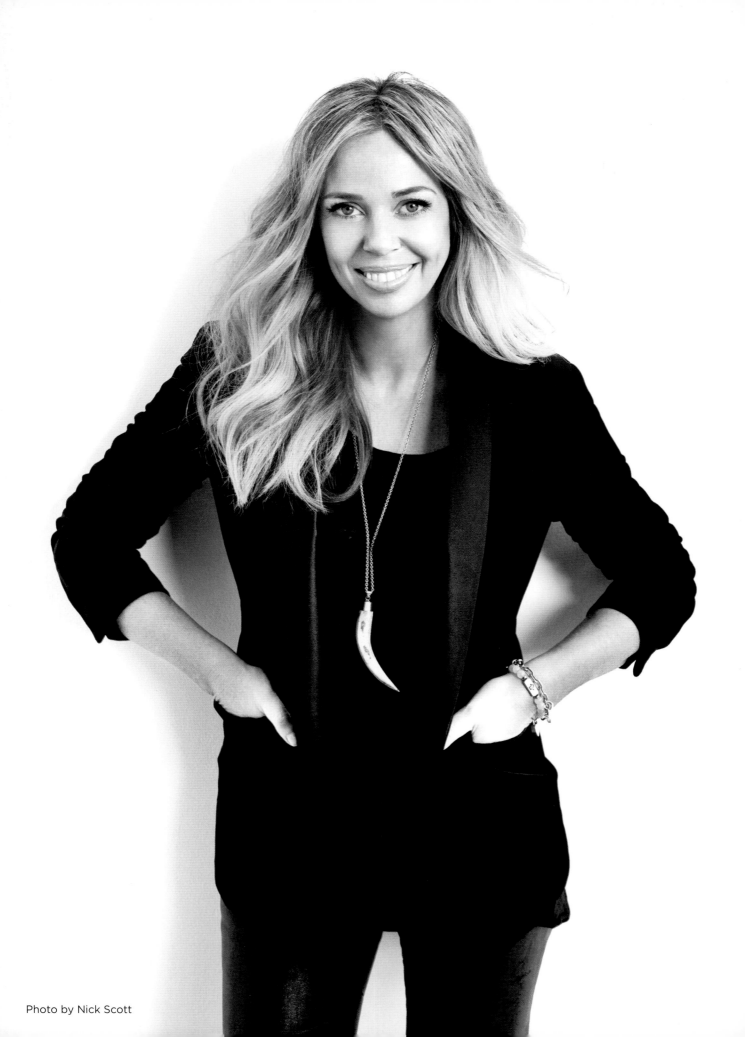

Afterword

Before I sign off, there's a few things I'd like to talk about. The most important thing is this: fashion is art. Every fashion image or runway show you see is the product of a whole team of people working to create that art. Every image you see has been retouched in some way — sometimes quite subtly, other times more dramatically. In fashion photography, there is technical retouching, where the levels of colours and dark and shade are adjusted, and then there's creative retouching, where the image is manipulated and changed. So while fashion is amazing and makes the world go round, the most important thing to remember is that the images should be seen as art. Take inspiration from the beauty campaigns and fashion magazines, but don't see them as something to copy.

This book isn't about hiding behind your makeup. It's about accepting yourself and enhancing what you've got. Makeup can transform you and help you feel more confident, so use it as a tool, start with a positive attitude and don't be afraid of it. Because that's the best thing about makeup — if you make a mistake, you can always take it off and do it again.

I know I'm more confident when I'm wearing makeup and I really hope this book gives you the skills to feel more confident too! Have fun!

Liz xxx

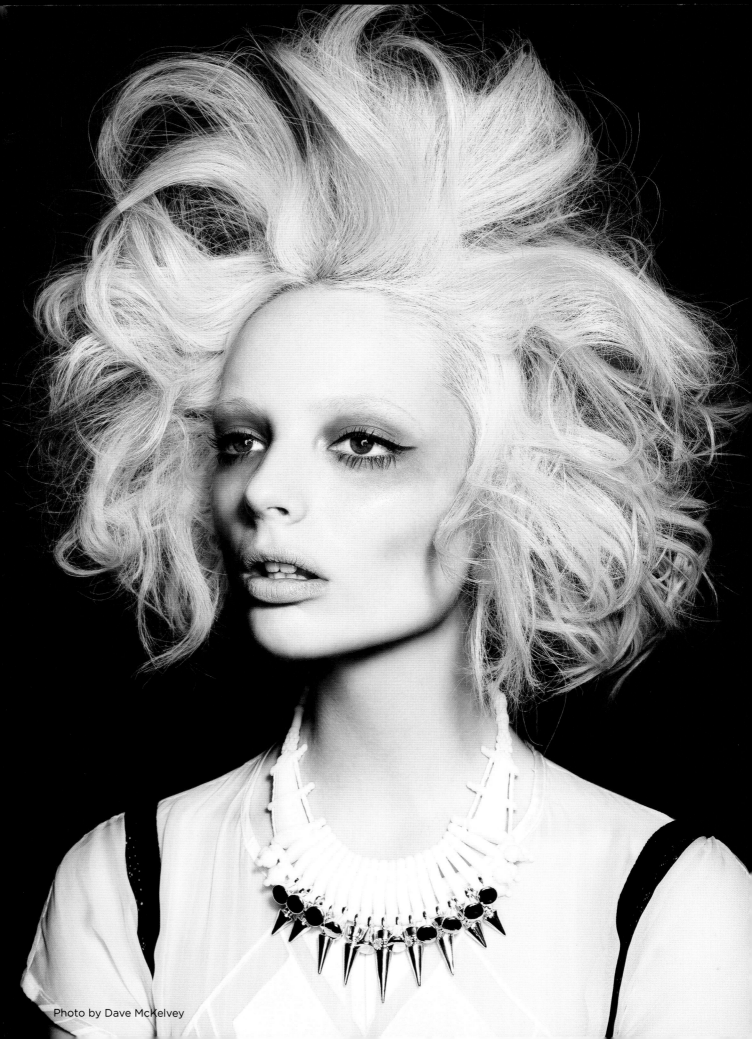

Photo by Dave McKelvey

Acknowledgements

This book wouldn't have been possible without the help of many people along the way. I love and thank them all.

My new and now dear friends at HarperCollins: Catherine Milne, my publisher, for her understanding and gently guiding this novice every step of the way. Editors Jennifer Blau, Rachel Dennis and Stephanie Darling for their magnificent nit-picking, which we love them for.

My awesome manager, Laura Mitchell, whose tenacity and patience rocks my world and makes rainbows appear.

My two superhero photographers, Steven Chee and Dave McKelvey, whose work (both new and archive) features vastly in this book, and who I drove bonkers and love dearly. One of the great things I love about my job is getting to work with talented artists like these two and I thank them from the bottom of my heart.

Photographer Milos Mlynarik for his kindness while shooting the Transformations chapter. Grace Testa for her delicate retouching. The many photographers, hairstylists and stylists whose work are in this book. Thank you.

And of course my strong, handsome and supportive husband, Dan, who always picks up the slack. Thank you for teaching Ava to read while I was writing.

Picture credits

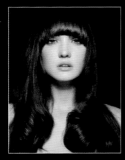

Image courtesy of *Harper's Bazaar* Australia, photographer Justin Cooper at 2c Management, model Sveva at Vivien's

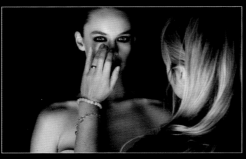

Image by Dave McKelvey; model Annabel at Chic Management

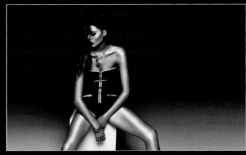

Image courtesy of valonz.com.au, photographer Dave McKelvey, model Gabby at Chic Management

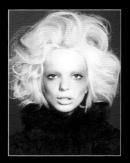

Image courtesy of valonz.com.au, photographer Dave McKelvey, model Chrystal at Chic Management

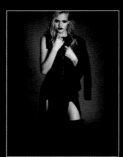

Image courtesy of Magdalena Velevska, photographer Liz Ham at 2c Management, model Rebecca at Work Agency

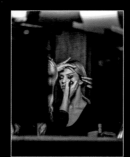

Image by Liz Kelsh, model Remy Green at Select Model Management

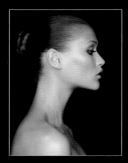

Image by Steven Chee at DLM, model Chloe at Priscilla's

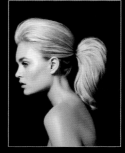

Image courtesy of *Harper's Bazaar* Australia, photographer Justin Cooper at 2c Management, model Jenny at Vivien's

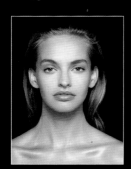

Image by Milos Mlynarik, model Janne at IMG Australia

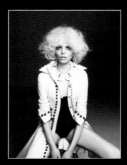

Image courtesy of valonz.com.au, photographer Dave McKelvey, model Chrystal at Chic Management

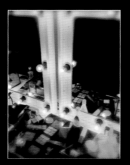

Image by Liz Kelsh

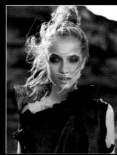

Image courtesy of valonz.com.au, photographer Dave McKelvey, model Tatyana at IMG Australia

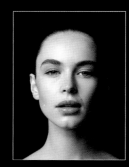

Image by Dave McKelvey, model Annabel at Chic Management

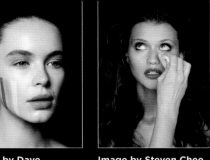

Image by Dave McKelvey, model Annabel at Chic Management

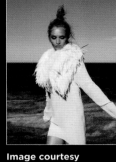

Image by Steven Chee at DLM, model Chloe at Priscilla's

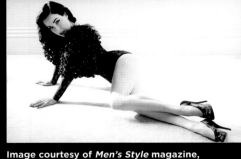

Image courtesy of valonz.com.au, photographer Dave McKelvey, model Tatyana at IMG Australia

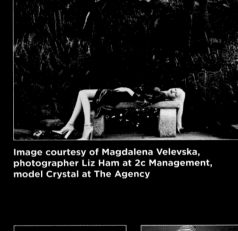

Image courtesy of Men's Style magazine, photographer Simon Lekias, featuring Dita Von Teese

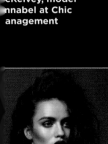

Image courtesy of valonz.com.au, photographer Dave McKelvey, model Gabby at Chic Mangaement

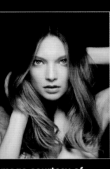

Image courtesy of Harper's Bazaar Australia, photographer Justin Cooper at 2c Management, model Jira at Chic Management

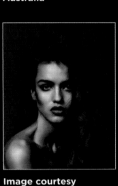

Image courtesy of valonz.com.au, photographer Dave McKelvey, model Gabby at Chic Management

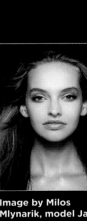

Image courtesy of Magdalena Velevska, photographer Liz Ham at 2c Management, model Crystal at The Agency

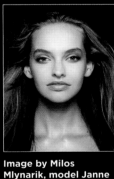

Image by Steven Chee at DLM, model Chloe at Priscilla's

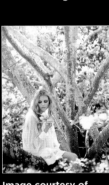

Image by Milos Mlynarik, model Janne at IMG Australia

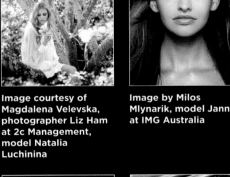

Image courtesy of Magdalena Velevska, photographer Liz Ham at 2c Management, model Natalia Luchinina

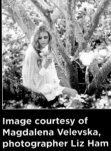

Image by Milos Mlynarik, model Janne at IMG Australia

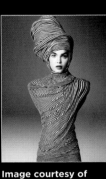

Image courtesy of Kirrilly Johnston, photographer Georges Antoni at The Artist Group, model Bambi at IMG Australia

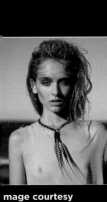

Image courtesy of valonz.com.au, photographer Dave McKelvey, model Tatyana at IMG

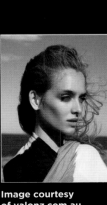

Image courtesy of valonz.com.au, photographer Dave McKelvey, model Tatyana at IMG

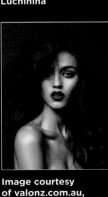

Image courtesy of valonz.com.au, photographer Dave McKelvey, model Gabby at Chic Management

Image courtesy of photographer Steven Chee at DLM, model Chloe at Priscilla's

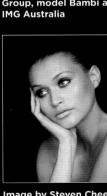

Image by Steven Chee at DLM, model Chloe at Priscilla's

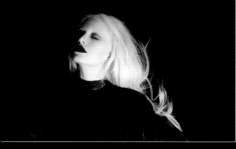

Image courtesy of Magdalena Velevska, photographer Liz Ham at 2c Management, model Crystal at The Agency

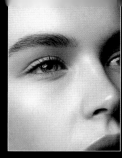

Image by Dave McKelvey, model Annabel at Chic Management

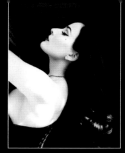

Image courtesy of *Men's Style* magazine, photographer Simon Lekias, featuring Dita Von Teese

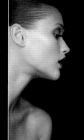

Image by Steven Chee at DLM, model Chloe at Priscilla's

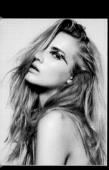

Image courtesy valonz.com.au, photographer Zachary Handley at The Artist Group, model Michon Chic Management

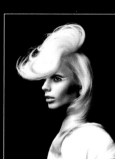

Image courtesy of valonz.com.au, photographer Dave McKelvey, model Chrystal at Chic Management

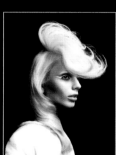

Image courtesy of valonz.com.au, photographer Dave McKelvey, model Chrystal at Chic Management

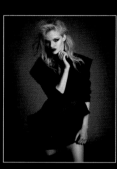

Image courtesy of Magdalena Velevska, photographer Liz Ham at 2c Mangement, model Rebecca at Work Agency

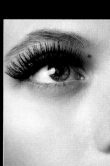

Image by Dave McKelvey, model Carly at Priscilla's

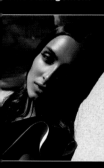

Image courtesy valonz.com.au, photographer Dave McKelvey, model tyana at IMG stralia

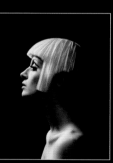

Image courtesy of valonz.com.au, photographer Dave McKelvey, model Ash Walker at Priscilla's

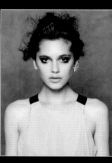

Image courtesy of valonz.com.au, photographer Zachary Handley at The Artist Group, model Anastasia at IMG Australia

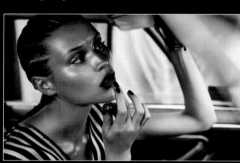

Image courtesy of photographer Steven Chee at DLM, model Chloe at Priscilla's

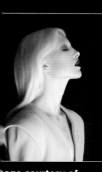

Image courtesy of Magdalena Velevska, photographer Liz Ham

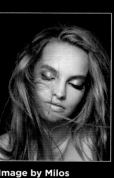

Image by Milos Mlynarik, model Janne at IMG Australia

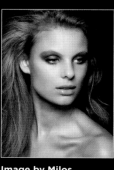

Image by Milos Mlynarik, model Ella Dieke at IMG Australia

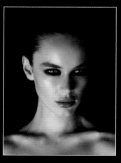

Image by Dave McKelvey, model Annabel at Chic

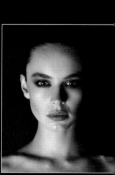

Image by Dave McKelvey, model Annabel at Chic

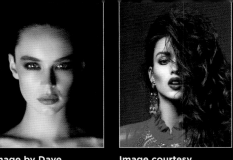
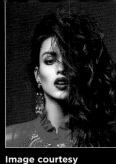
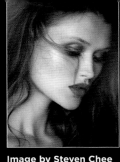
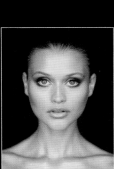
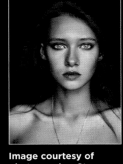
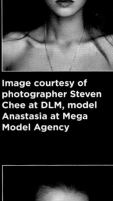
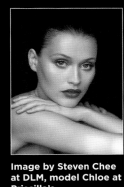
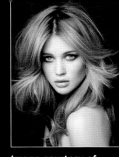

Image by Dave cKelvey, model nnabel at Chic anagement

Image courtesy of valonz.com.au, photographer Dave McKelvey, model Gabby at Chic Management

Image by Steven Chee at DLM, model Chloe at Priscilla's

Image courtesy of photographer Steven Chee at DLM, model Anastasia at Mega Model Agency

Image courtesy of *Harper's Bazaar* Australia, photographe Justin Cooper at 2c Management, model Scherri-Lee at Vivien's

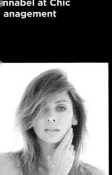
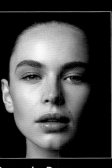
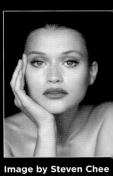
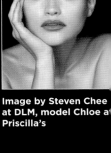

Image courtesy of ailis, photographer ierre Toussaint, eaturing Natalie mbruglia

Image by Dave McKelvey, model Annabel at Chic Mangement

Image by Steven Chee at DLM, model Chloe at Priscilla's

Image by Steven Chee at DLM, model Chloe at Priscilla's

Image by Steven Chee at DLM, model Chloe at Priscilla's

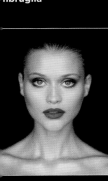
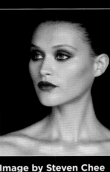
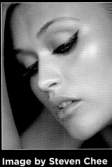
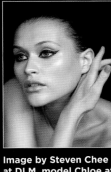
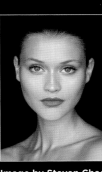

Image by Steven Chee t DLM, model Chloe at riscilla's

Image by Steven Chee at DLM, model Chloe at Priscilla's

Image by Steven Chee at DLM, model Chloe at Priscilla's

Image by Steven Chee at DLM, model Chloe at Priscilla's

Image by Steven Chee at DLM, model Chloe a Priscilla's

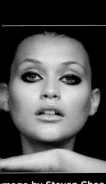
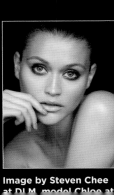
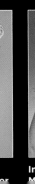
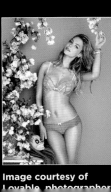
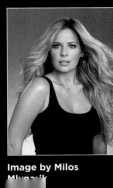
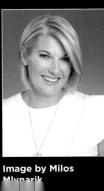

Image by Steven Chee t DLM, model Chloe at

Image by Steven Chee at DLM, model Chloe at

Image courtesy of Lovable, photographer

Image by Milos Mlynarik

Image by Milos Mlynarik

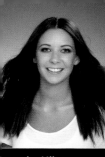

Image by Milos Mlynarik

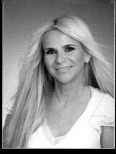

Image by Milos Mlynarik

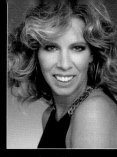

Image by Milos Mlynarik

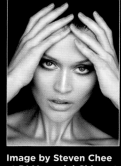

Image by Steven Chee at DLM, model Chloe at Priscilla's

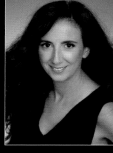

Image by Milos Mlynarik

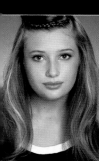

Image by Milos Mlynarik

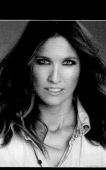

Image by Milos Mlynarik

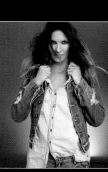

Image by Milos Mlynarik

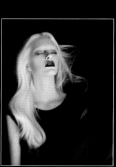

Image courtesy of Magdalena Velaveska, photographer Liz Ham at 2c Mangement, model Crystal at The Agency

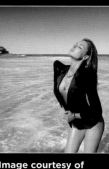

Image courtesy of *Harper's Bazaar* Australia, photographer Georges Antoni at The Artist Group, featuring Jennifer Hawkins

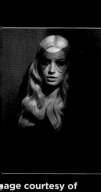

Image courtesy of *Harper's Bazaar* Australia, photographer m Haskins, model nya at Vivien's

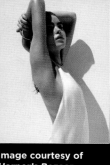

Image courtesy of *Harper's Bazaar* Australia, photographer Pierre Toussaint, model Bambi at IMG Australia

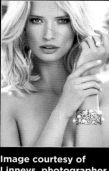

Image courtesy of Linneys, photographer Nick Leary, model Jessica van der Steen at Models 1

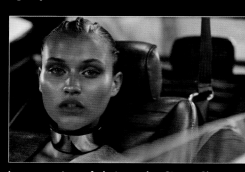

Image courtesy of photographer Steven Chee at DLM, model Chloe at Priscilla's

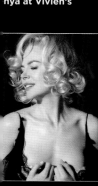

age courtesy of rper's Bazaar stralia, photographer

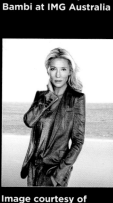

Image courtesy of *Vogue*, photographer Steven Chee, featuring

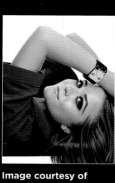

Image courtesy of *Harper's Bazaar* Australia, photographer

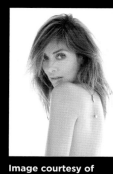

Image courtesy of Kailis, photographer Pierre Toussaint,

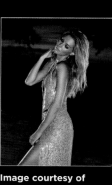

Image courtesy of Jbronze, photographer Steven Chee at DLM,

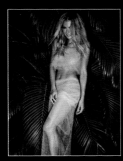

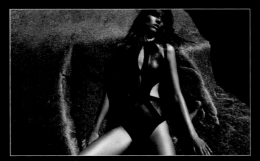

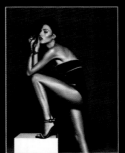

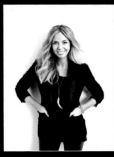

Image courtesy of Jbronze, photographer Steven Chee at DLM, featuring Jennifer Hawkins

Image courtesy of valonz.com.au, photographer Dave McKelvey, model Tatyana at IMG Australia

Image courtesy of valonz.com.au, photographer Dave McKelvey, model Gabby at Chic Management

Image courtesy of Bauer Media Pty Ltd, photographer Nick Scott

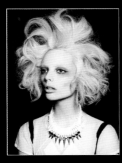

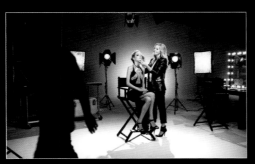

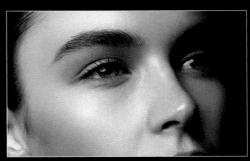

Image courtesy of valonz.com.au, photographer Dave McKelvey, model Chrystal at Chic Management

Image courtesy of Max Factor, photographer Milos Mlynarik, model Tatyana at IMG Australia

Image by Dave McKelvey, model Annabel at Chic Management

Drawings of face and eyes template by Kerrie Hess, makeup by Liz Kelsh

Drawings of brushes on pages 26–7, lashes on pages 96–7 and colour wheel on page 203 by Hazel Lam, HarperCollins Design Studio

Images on pages 210–1 courtesy of Liz Kelsh

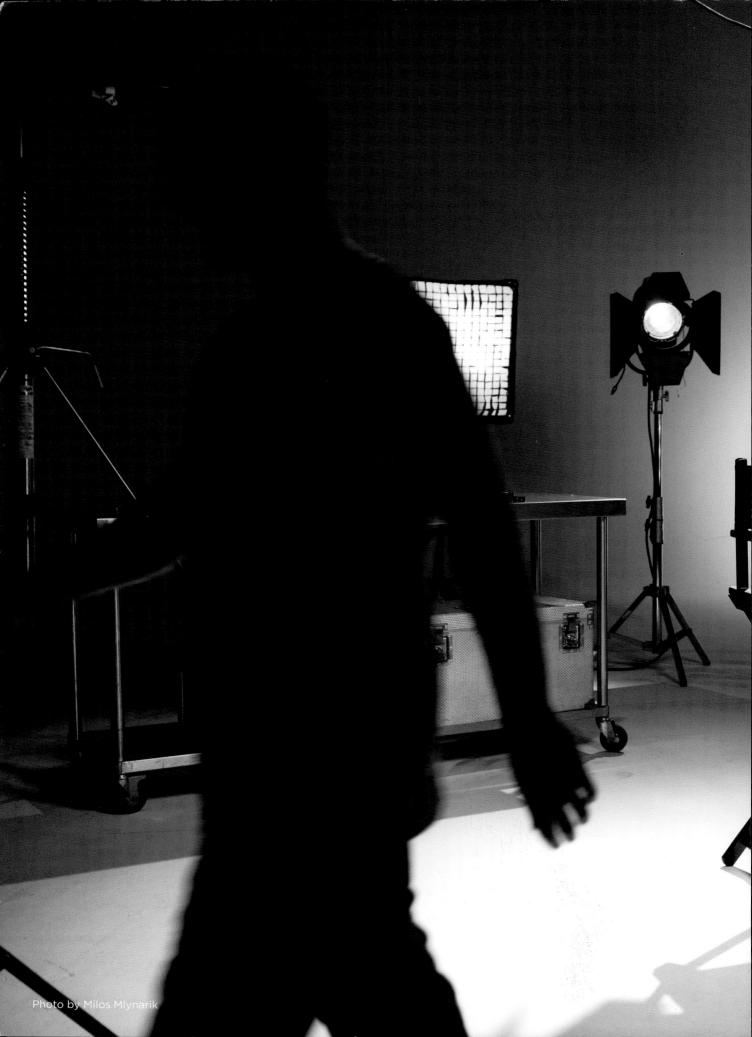

Photo by Milos Mlynarik

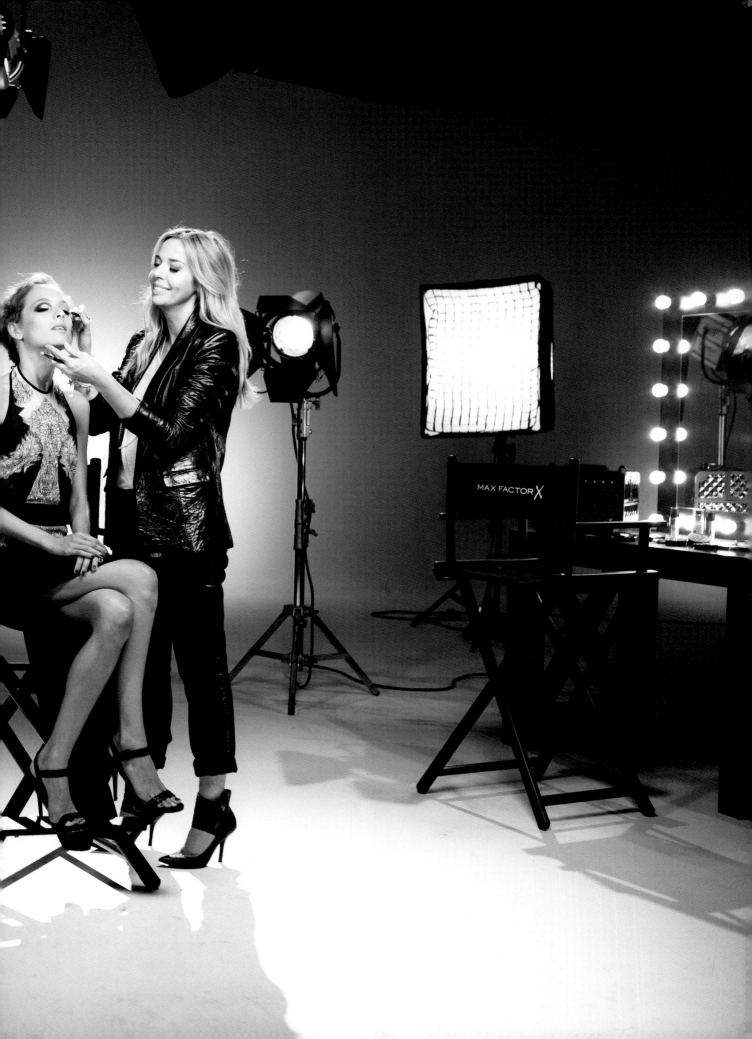

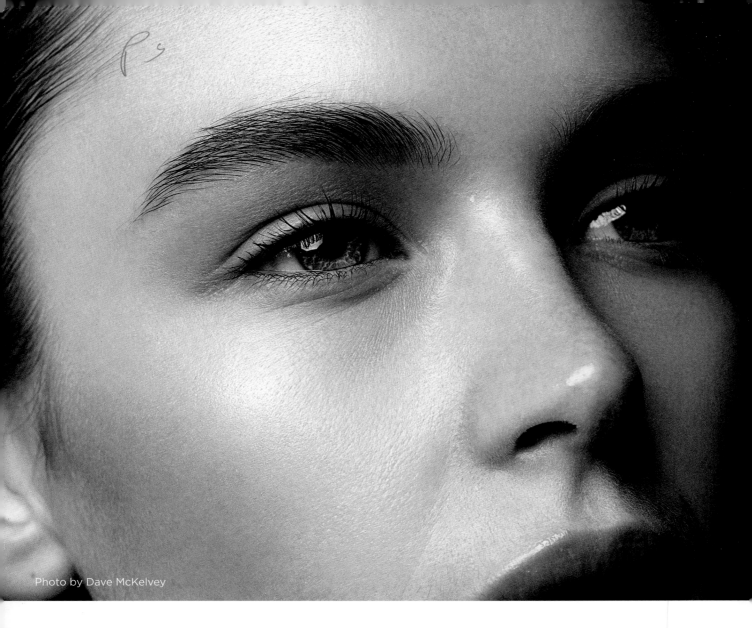

Photo by Dave McKelvey

HarperCollins*Publishers*

First published in Australia in 2014
by HarperCollins*Publishers* Australia Pty Limited
ABN 36 009 913 517
harpercollins.com.au

Text copyright © Liz Kelsh 2014

HarperCollins*Publishers*
Level 13, 201 Elizabeth Street, Sydney, NSW 2000, Australia
Unit D1, 63 Apollo Drive, Rosedale, Auckland 0632, New Zealand
A 53, Sector 57, Noida, UP, India
77–85 Fulham Palace Road, London W6 8JB, United Kingdom
2 Bloor Street East, 20th floor, Toronto, Ontario M4W 1A8, Canada
195 Broadway, New York, NY 10007, USA

National Library of Australia Cataloguing-in-Publication data:

Kelsh, Liz.
    Makeup by Liz Kelsh / Liz Kelsh.
    978 0 7322 9800 5 (pbk.)
    Beauty, Personal — Popular works
    Cosmetics — Popular works
391.63

Cover and internal design by Hazel Lam,
HarperCollins Design Studio
Cover photographs by Steven Chee
Author photograph by Nick Scott/Bauer Media Pty Ltd
Edited by Stephanie Darling
Layout and typesetting by Kate Barraclough,
Kate Frances Design
Colour reproduction by Graphic Print Group, Adelaide
Printed and bound in China by RR Donnelley on 128gsm matt art